D1011092

THE COMING
CANCER
BREAKTHROUGHS

THE COMING CANCER BREAKTHROUGHS

▼

What You Need to Know About the Latest Cancer Treatment Options

JOSEPH F. DOOLEY, Ph.D., F.A.C.B., and MARIAN BETANCOURT

KENSINGTON BOOKS
http://www.kensingtonbooks.com

This book presents information based upon the research and personal experiences of the authors. It is not intended to be a substitute for a professional consultation with a physician or other health-care provider. Neither the publisher nor the authors can be held responsible for any adverse effects or consequences resulting from the use of any of the information in this book. They also cannot be held responsible for any errors or omissions in the book. If you have a condition that requires medical advice, the publisher and authors urge you to consult a competent health-care professional.

This book is dedicated to the memory of my mother, Dorothy Dooley, who fought a valiant battle against breast cancer for several years, but ultimately died from it. This was long before biochemistry and medicine could help her. Now patients with this disease have a chance to live. It was through her lifelong support and encouragement that this book was formed.

—J.D.

For the millions of us who have confronted cancer and survived and for the millions more who are yet to meet this challenge, this book is for you.

—M.B.

Contents

Acknowledgments

It would be impossible to name and thank all of the people who gave so generously of their time and expertise to help in the formation of this book. They include patients, doctors and scientists, and others who work in the biotech industry. However, special thanks go to Garo Armen, Ph.D., and Jonathan Lewis, M.D., Ph.D., at Antigenics; Dr. Sam Waskal, Andrea Rabney, John Landes, and Nick Giorgio, Ph.D., at ImClone; Dr. Wornell at Genta; Dr. Henny at Dendreon; Jacqueline Johnson, Ph.D., at FeRx; Elaine Orenberg, Ph.D., at Matrix Pharmaceutical, Inc.; Carlyn Wickens, M.D., at Immunomedics, Inc.; A. Lisa Self, Pharm.D., at InterMune Pharmaceuticals; and Neil Berinstein, M.D., at Aventis Corporation.

To those at hospitals and medical centers, appreciation and thanks to Waun Ki Hong, M.D., and Fadlo Kjhuri, M.D., at the M. D. Anderson Cancer Center; Daniel Hayes, M.D., Lombardi Cancer Center, Georgetown University Medical Center; Larry Norton, M.D., Memorial Sloan-Kettering Cancer Center and president, American Society of Clinical Oncology; Howard Hochster, M.D., associate professor of clinical medicine, New York University School of Medicine; and Lawrence Einhorn, M.D., past president of the American Society of Clinical Oncology.

In addition, a thank-you to the Honorable Nancy L. Johnson,

representative, United States Congress, and Nancy Goodman Brinker of the Susan G. Komen Breast Cancer Foundation.

We would also like to acknowledge the dedication of editors Claire Gerus and Elaine Will Sparber and literary agent Vicky Bijur for making this book possible.

But most especially, we want to acknowledge the tireless and valuable help and support of Joyce Kuhn to Dr. Dooley during the formation of this book.

Preface

Early in the 20th century, medical researchers learned that cancer could be induced in animals by exposure to many different types of chemicals. In the 1950s and 1960s they had begun to understand that the cancer process can start early in life and not show up as clinical disease until years later. This was the situation in cancer research up until a few years ago. It was a valiant battle fought by researchers, physicians, and patients. Sometimes there were moments of triumph, but more often than most oncologists would care to admit, defeat and death were the inevitable outcome. Technology and the mapping of the human genome have changed everything. We've moved from test tubes to microchips. This is a paradigm shift in research.

The standard treatment for cancer had always been surgery or, if that was not feasible because of the location of the tumor, then chemotherapy or radiation. These terrible treatments worked, at least to some extent. Some patients survived their initial bout with the disease. But too many times patients would be condemned to undergo long-term therapy that destroyed their quality of life only to succumb in the end. Family members who witnessed the treatments often wondered whether the cure was worse than the disease. Worst of all, the long-term cure rate for the most deadly types of cancer, like lung or pancreatic cancer, had not gone down significantly in years. Clearly another approach must be tried. By the end of the 20th century that new approach was on the horizon.

At a 1998 biotech conference in New York City the excitement was palpable. Top scientists and leaders of companies engaging in biotechnology research around the world—over 2,000 of them—were there. Only about 3 percent of the human genome had been decoded, but already scientists were beginning to understand how cancer really works at the level of DNA. Two years later, at the start of the 21st century, the genome was completed.

There was very little of the usual hype we had heard in the past: A new technique is discovered. A few promising leads are followed, and then we see it reported on the evening news. Millions of people have their expectations of a cancer cure raised, thousands of letters pour into the research centers mentioned in the report, and then nothing. Just another premature research report. A few good results in mice. No effective results in people. The truth is that cancer was cured years ago in mice. In fact, the director of the National Cancer Institute (NCI) was quoted recently as saying that "the history of cancer research is about curing cancer in the mouse." That's not the problem. Bringing the promise of good research ideas from the test tube or the mouse to people—that's the problem. For decades now the progress has been excruciatingly slow. But no more. This time the DNA approach seems to work in people.

Still, the investigators and executives at the 1998 meeting were cautious. It was as if they did not want to go through all of the hyperbole again. They saw exciting results and talked to each other about the new possibilities, but to the press and the public they were mute. They didn't want to raise any false hopes.

All that changed three years later at the 2001 annual meeting of the American Society of Clinical Oncology. At this superbowl of cancer research meetings, even more astounding news was revealed. And the investigators and everybody else were no longer so silent. More than 25,000 oncologists were overflowing meeting rooms and hallways in San Francisco, discussing the latest and most promising cancer treatments. At this meeting we learned there really was a magic bullet—at least one for a form of leukemia. The success of Gleevec, a targeted monoclonal antibody, was front-page news around the world. And it brought incredible hope and encouragement to the people creating these new therapies as well as the people who will now benefit from them.

During those three years, I followed these ideas and interviewed scores of people involved in this exciting new research and cancer treatment. As a biochemist I was able to speak their language, and as a person who had lost a loved one to cancer, I was well aware of the emotional urgency of these new developments. I interviewed doctors involved in clinical studies with these new therapies. I spoke with patients who had gained hope for many more years of life from this cutting-edge treatment. Their stories are here, but I have changed their names to protect their privacy.

Joseph Dooley, Ph.D., F.A.C.B.

INTRODUCTION

A bipartisan national poll during the 2000 presidential election revealed that Americans care more about finding a cure for cancer than they do about nuclear missile defense, violent crime, environmental protection, or campaign finance reform. Finding a cure for cancer ranked second only to providing health care to all children on a list of goals America should set for the future. The poll was commissioned by a small group of nationally recognized cancer survivors and scientists that included Lance Armstrong and his oncologist, Dr. Craig Nichols; Hamilton Jordan; and Nobel Laureate Dr. Phillip A. Sharp, in collaboration with the American Association for Cancer Research (AACR).

Cancer touches the lives of most Americans; 73 percent have had a close friend or family member die of the disease, and 45 percent say they know someone who had cancer and was cured. You'll meet some of those people in this book, including many of the leaders of the biotech drug research who were set on their path because of a personal involvement in cancer. Cancer touched my life, too, and that's what prompted this book. My mother died of breast cancer. She was treated at one of the leading university centers in the country. She had a career in medicine management. I was a biochemist involved in cancer research. We had access to all the latest treatments. My mother had a lumpectomy, a procedure that removes the cancerous lesion from the breast but does not disfigure the woman as a mastectomy would. The technique was new then, but over the years it has proved to be the surgery of choice. My mother and I made all the right decisions for her care.

Five years had passed, and we thought that she had successfully conquered cancer. We were terribly wrong. All the positive plans, all the love, all the good habits like not ever smoking, eating nutritiously, and getting regular exercise meant nothing. The cancer had come back just as perniciously as it had come the first time, this time in her brain.

The doctors turned loose their full armamentarium. They gave my mother toxic drugs that were supposed to kill the tumor. But the treatment only made her sicker. They put her in a giant X-ray machine, one that would scare any healthy young person. But my mother was 64 and very ill. They bombarded her with ionizing radiation in an attempt to kill the tumor in her brain. The result was only that she lost the ability to talk and to walk.

Mercifully, the last days of my mother's life were spent in a coma. I stayed with her almost every moment. She had given me life, and now I watched her life slowly being squeezed out of her by the relentless growth of the tumor. The doctors couldn't do anything for her, I thought, but they were using techniques that were decades old, terribly dangerous and toxic, and of little real use anyway. I had studied this disease professionally and knew all about the current research, yet I was helpless to do anything but stand there and watch my mother die.

This book is about where we are now, at the beginning of the 21st century. However, the book must be more than a report of the magnificent advances in sciences and biotechnology of the last five years. That's an interesting subject, but it's not going to directly help anybody.

It's also important that this book not be simply a dry compendium of drugs for cancer. That wouldn't help anybody either. No, in order to reach the most people, and put exciting science and terrible diseases into a place where the reader can grasp the important points and move closer to therapeutic success, this book must tell the story of the fight against cancer. It must tell of the individual scientists and doctors who are dedicated to finding lasting therapeutic answers. It must tell of the new ways that biotechnology is approaching this old scourge of mankind.

Here we name names, give company information, and list addresses and telephone numbers of places to go to find new therapies for cancer. Here we explain as clearly as possible what the idea is behind these new drug therapies. Here we will try to give hope to cancer patients who have already been through the cancer mill and still find themselves in a life-threatening place.

In the next few years there will be many very effective treatments for all types of cancer. Cancer will be treated much more like a serious but chronic condition like heart disease. Drug therapies will be effective in regressing tumors but will not have the draconian side effects of the present standard treatments of toxic drugs and radiation. Patients will be able to take medicines orally, at home, under a doctor's general care for long periods, even a lifetime, to produce effective remissions of disease. The combination of early diagnosis coupled with molecular target therapeutics will provide long-term survival rates above 90 percent for a wide variety of cancers.

In this book you will find a balanced view of the new approaches to cancer therapy. You'll find information that might give hope for a successful outcome to someone struggling with cancer. If you or a family member has been newly diagnosed with cancer, this book will help you better understand new cutting-edge therapeutic approaches and make more informed choices with your doctor. It contains specific information about the latest treatments for different types of cancer, the medical centers that provide the best treatment, lists of ongoing clinical trials, and phone numbers and web sites of the companies that are providing new therapies. You will be able to find out where the clinical research centers are, and the names of the physicians running the trials.

It is important to understand that there is no magic bullet to "cure" cancer. Cancer therapy has been developing gradually by trial and error for the last 50 years. Traditional approaches do work in some cases. John Wayne lived for 25 years after his first operation for lung cancer. He made a lot of movies during that time. It is critical that people who are diagnosed with cancer seek out and find an experienced oncologist who is expert at dealing with their form of cancer. To do otherwise would be foolish and life-threatening. After all, when my own mother was diagnosed with cancer, we sought out the best physicians that we could find.

But it is equally important when confronted by a life-threatening disease to ask the right questions. An informed person must ask: What about the new techniques that are just being developed for cancer? Should they be considered in my form of cancer? Where are the trials being held? Is my doctor or hospital involved?

Learn all that you can about your disease and be willing to go the extra mile to find out what the right treatment is for you. This is even truer if you have advanced cancer. Maybe surgery is simply not enough to take care of the problem. Standard treatments might not be enough anymore. So don't give up. Fight! And look for new therapies that may be right for you.

Cancer therapy will always be a mixture of art and science. Because of the complex nature of the disease, it will always borrow from the traditional treatments as well as the cutting-edge approaches.

There is a sea change in understanding of how cancer works and how to stop it. And that is worth hoping for.

Everyone deals with cancer in a different way. I hope that the descriptions of exciting new scientific advances that appear in this book will give you cause for courage in the face of fear. I believe that this information will empower you to seek out the best treatment. As David G. Nance, president and CEO of Introgen Therapeutics, Inc., a privately held Austin, Texas, biotech company, told that group of researchers gathered at the New York Sheraton in 1998, "If I were cancer right now, I'd be damned worried."

Joseph Dooley, Ph.D., F.A.C.B.

PART ONE

▼

UNDERSTANDING OUR BIOMOLECULAR SELVES

CHAPTER 1

▼

MICROANATOMY
The Body's Software

Did you ever walk down the street in a large city like Chicago or New York and wonder how there could be so many different designs for people who are basically the same? The billions of people on earth all need the same air to breathe; the same glucose fuels their cells, and the same heartbeats push the same hemoglobin around their bodies. And yet we all are so incredibly different. We have different fingerprints, different heights and shapes, different voices and skin colors. Our facial features are the same—with eyes, nose, mouth—yet they are all different. We are different but yet the same because of the human genome.

Five years ago no one had ever heard of the human genome, except for a few bioresearch scientists. It's long and complicated, like an engineering manual or a dry doctoral thesis, but it is also the map of our lives. Every one of the trillions of cells in our bodies contains a copy of this long ribbonlike instruction sheet. It is composed of billions of "letters" of DNA (deoxyribonucleic acid) encoding 30,000 individual genes. All human beings possess this incredible biochemical master list that controls every process in our bodies. Without it we could not live. Indeed, without it we would not be human.

Humans have the highest number of individual genes of any animal on earth. We are by far the most complicated beings around, although we don't really know who else may be out there in the universe.

The 30,000 genes and the billion or so DNA letters can be varied in many ways. On top of this is the fact that most of our traits like the ability to digest foods, susceptibility to diseases, and life span are the result of the interaction of many different genes acting in sequence. So you can see that the basic design we call human beings can be varied in literally tens of billions of ways. We are far more complex than computers.

MUTATIONS: A GLITCH IN THE COPY MACHINE

But any system this complex must have errors. These errors are called mutations. No, they're not absurd Hollywood monsters or Mutant Ninja Turtles. Mutations are changes in the DNA spelling. During DNA synthesis, which is controlled by the genes, thousands of pairs are made each minute in the nucleus of the cell. This process goes on all the time. This is how our bodies operate at the molecular level. Well, it's natural to suspect that a certain rate of error will occur in linking up these pairs, much as a knitting machine will make an occasional error when threading yarn together into a complex pattern. This is just what happens in our cells.

A very low error rate in forming DNA results in an occasional bad copy. The body screens for this just the way a factory quality-control inspector checks the pattern in the cloth being woven. The same is true for a DNA mistake. It doesn't fit right and the cell removes it. Little harm is done. More good copies are immediately made.

But what if the mistake is not so obvious? What if the change in the DNA coding, the mutation, was so subtle that the body didn't recognize it? Maybe nothing important would happen. Maybe that particular DNA would cause a small malfunction in a cell and the cell would die. No problem. We have trillions of cells. And even in important areas like the liver or the brain, the loss of one or two, or even thousands, of cells would not be noticed.

ALTERED STATES

However, if the cell doesn't die, but lives on in some altered state that changes its function, then what happens? And what if many thousands of cells became altered in the same way? This is a lot of "what if's." But it happens to all of us routinely. We call it aging. When a skin cell is altered, perhaps it cannot excrete the right mixture of oils, so our skin texture changes. Maybe an elastin cell doesn't quite work anymore, so a wrinkle in the skin appears. Maybe there's a change in melatonin metabolism in certain skin cells, and we see aging spots. It happens all through life, until the cumulative process of change overtakes our bodies, and we die of old age. (There is no programming for how long we will live. While longevity is increasing, our individual longevity depends on us.)

But maybe a more insidious change in the DNA blueprint occurs. Maybe there is a change that does not kill the cell but in fact liberates it, makes it immortal so to speak. It becomes a terrorist or renegade in our body. That cell escapes the body's normal growth controls. It begins to multiply again and again. Probably this change in growth pattern is accompanied by some change in function, or more likely, after a while there are just too many of this one type of cell—just as an airplane couldn't function properly if there were five times more passengers aboard than the plane was designed to hold. We call this uncontrolled growth of one of our cells "cancer."

All cancers start somewhere, sometime. Unlike bacterial infections, which start after an exposure to many millions of microorganisms at once, or like chronic diseases such as diabetes or arteriosclerosis, which start after a long sequence of metabolic changes, cancer starts always with one specific cell in one particular place.

Depending on the cell type, a new cancer cell may take years or even decades to develop into a cellular mass of 10,000 cells weighing about 100 grams—the size of your thumb—the stage where a tumor is clinically noticeable. The DNA may have changed 30 years ago, but the "cancer" is showing up now. This is the problem with cancer in a nutshell.

Since every cancer starts from a single cell, it takes a relatively long time to build up against the body's very formidable defenses, sometimes years. Some cancer cells grow and spread faster than others as well, and this growth rate can often be measured. Until that time they are for the most part silent, unless you're lucky enough to have one near a nerve or on the surface of your skin where it is more likely to be detected.

CELLS ARE US

The cells that we call cancer have proven themselves to be very adaptable and very viable. They are us. They are not strangers introduced from the outside. The cancer cells when they appear in our bodies are of the same substance as the rest of our cells, and they most likely have had years to grow and become successful.

We know cancer is a complex group of diseases characterized by uncontrolled proliferation of abnormal cells. This uncontrolled growth is often caused by genetic defects or mutations. These may be a result of an inherited tendency, or they may be the result of some insult from the environment, or lifestyle factors like smoking. Or they could simply be from random errors in DNA replication as cells normally grow and divide. Some tissues in our bodies, such as the digestive tract, shed and replace tens of millions of cells every day. It's no wonder that sometimes mistakes can be made.

When a single cell amasses a number of mutations, usually over a period of years, and the normal restraints on proliferation no longer apply, cancer starts. That cell and its descendants continue to mutate and accumulate to form a tumor made up primarily of these abnormal cells. The primary danger of malignancies (cancer cells or tumors) is that they can migrate (metastasize) and carry the disease to other parts of the body.

Because the cancer cells have been there so long, getting them all out with surgery is very difficult. Theoretically, if even one cell manages to evade the surgeon's knife, the disease will recur. However, since most human cancers are relatively slow-growing, you may be able to outlive the cancer if the whole process of cancer growth is pushed back to square one by surgical removal of most of the cells.

The other therapeutic approaches to cancer involve radiation or toxic drugs. The problem is that the cancer cells are so much like normal cells that these forms of treatment will kill all cell types indiscriminately. So doctors rely on stratagems that will protect most of the "good" cells and kill most of the "bad" ones. It sometimes works, thank goodness, but it is crude. It's sort of like using a blowtorch inside a house to kill termites. The bugs die, but so does the house. The current medical approach is to kill as many bugs as possible without burning the house to the ground. It doesn't always work.

TINKERING WITH THE BLUEPRINT

Now, however, a new way of looking at this problem has been uncovered. Since all cancers originate by changes in the cell's master blueprint, the gene, then it might be possible to base cancer therapy on these changes in the cell. Treatments that target the cancer cell's own DNA would selectively target abnormal cells and leave normal cells alone. Not only would there be an opportunity to seek and destroy all of the cancer cells in the patient, but there would be none of the toxic side effects that now limit the usefulness of therapy.

The DNA uses the stored information in the genes to instruct the cell to make proteins, which are the building blocks of the cell. In order to make the cell work right, the genetic information is used to make proteins necessary for cell life. Different genes give different proteins. So structural components come from one set of genes; other biological processes come from another set of genes. It's much like building and running a house. The carpenters use one set of instructions to build the walls and the roof. The electricians use a different set of instructions to wire the house for electricity and power. And the cook in the kitchen uses still a different set to bake the bread, in an oven that uses electricity and sits next to the kitchen wall.

Our bodies have evolved over tens of millions of years. They are finely tuned biological machines. We have seen how they are run by the instructions in DNA. The proteins that are made from the DNA blueprint are manufactured in our cells at rates of thousands of copies per second. The best, most advanced factories in the world, with all of the most complex computer programs, couldn't match that. And we don't even think about it.

As the years go along, there are inevitable mistakes in the formation of these proteins. But even the smallest error rate of 0.0001 percent can produce a number of mistakes in a lifetime of making new proteins. The big mistakes are usually of little consequence. They are so defective that they don't work at all. The body quickly destroys these copies and makes new ones. It has a host of protective mechanisms for just such occasions.

LITTLE MISTAKES, BIG PROBLEMS

It's the little mistakes that become a problem. They are not enough to totally compromise the function of newly created proteins, but they do interfere. The result is that these slightly defective building blocks get used by the body. But they don't work quite right. We recognize this problem as aging. Our skin becomes thinner and less supple. Our ears don't hear as sharply. Our joints and tendons are stiffer. We get wrinkles. These parts of our bodies usually work, but not as well as they did when they were new and young and all the proteins were just right.

Well, the same thing happens to the blueprints. After all, they are just proteins, just parts of the body that have to be continually remade and replaced. But when the blueprints get themselves wrong, all the other parts that depend on their instructions go wrong as well. And there is the basis of cancer.

When the DNA is changed, or mutated, either by a chance mistake in the synthesis or by an errant cosmic ray, the cell which depends on that DNA to give it instructions changes, too. If the change is a big one, the cell cannot survive, and it dies. Since there are billions of cells in our bodies, and every vital organ system has millions of cells, this is not a big problem. In fact, it's good. A dead cell is quickly destroyed by the body's killer T cells and disposed of safely. It's a natural part of the life cycle, and we are designed by that 10-million-year history to handle it quite well.

But when there's a mistake that is not fatal to the cell, but changes it in certain ways, there can be trouble—big trouble. Some changes in the DNA result in cells' losing their ability to control growth. They become immortal. They escape the natural ebb and flow of the body's turnover. They divide and confer this out-of-control growth to daughter cells, which become a growing army of terrorists. This process of division continues unchecked over hundreds of generations of cells. The result is the disease we know as cancer.

Since all cancers start with one cell at some very specific moment, and don't progress to the clinical disease of cancer until they start interfering with the body's natural functions, it may take years or even decades for a change like this to be a problem. This is why cancers of very active tissues like the breast, ovaries, or colon are so common. The cell turnover in these tissues is high, and therefore the cancers grow faster. In other tissues like the tendons, the muscles, or the heart, cell turnover is low, so cancers of these organs, although they do occur, are a lot less common.

The point of all this is to recognize that there is a built-in predisposition to cancer in our cells. The process that leads to cancer in our bodies is a natural thing. It occurs in all other animals that have a long life. If we are around long enough, it will probably happen to all of us, too.

THE BODY'S NATIONAL GUARD

The situation is not as bleak as it looks at first glance. Of course, there is a chance of cellular mistakes that lead to cancer. That's the way our bodies are made. But our bodies also have ample means to fight cancer and defeat it. We have evolved an immune system not only to fight outside threats to our biological well-being, but also to protect us from the dangers that come from within.

Our bodies contain special cells called killer T cells that specialize in circulating through the body and seeking out cells that are defective. When these degenerate cells are identified, they are quickly overcome and destroyed. So there are some natural protections.

Of course, mankind has also found some very specific drugs that kill cancer cells. These form the basis of current treatments of chemotherapy. The trouble is that these drugs are toxic to normal, good cells as well. They are also very nonspecific. Doctors have to give large amounts of these toxic substances in order to kill the cancer cells. But in doing so, a lot of normal cells get killed, too. That's the reason many chemotherapy regimens have such severe side effects.

But now we have a different approach. Instead of bombing the body with showers of toxic drugs in an attempt to kill everything in sight—friend or foe—biotechnology has begun to use what is known about cancer genetics to fashion exquisite new tools like gene therapy, monoclonal antibodies, cancer vaccines, and angiogenesis inhibitors.

We have seen that now, at the beginning of the 21st century, after 40 years of "the war on cancer," we can reasonably expect, using science, to successfully fight this disease. But there is more.

We now understand an enormous amount about how cancers work at the cellular level to cause disease. In the human genome project, we are just beginning to catalog the DNA blueprint that all of the cells in our bodies use. In the not too distant future, we will be in a position to put these two pieces of knowledge together.

Since all cancers start with one single cell, and all of the cells in a cancerous tumor have the same DNA, it follows that if we can identify the specific change in the cancer DNA, we will have the cause of the tumor.

But more than that: if we can know what has changed in a cell to make it a cancer cell, then we might be able to understand what changes to make to stop the cancer cell from growing uncontrollably, or kill it and its progeny altogether. In other words, cancer could be treated at the level of DNA. It could be turned off, or eliminated. And only those cells that were cancerous would be affected. All the hundreds of millions of normal cells that the body uses every minute for life would be spared.

This is not a dream. Once scientists learn what the DNA sequence is in normal cells, then they can look at cancer cells. They can ask the question, what is the difference between these two cells? Why is the cancer cell different? What is the change in the DNA? Knowing what the specific problem is for each type of cancer, and there will be different solutions for different cancers, they can set about to fix what's broken.

This is a lot like how I used to fix my old Chevrolet when I was in college. It was always breaking down; usually an aging part in the engine would give out, and my car would malfunction. Well, I couldn't afford to take the car to a mechanic every time it had trouble. The solution: I asked my friend Danny, who had the same model of Chevy, to help me. We located the source of the problem by comparing the parts of each engine until we found the part that wasn't working. Then we replaced that one part, and sure enough, the car ran again—until the next time.

We didn't rip out half of the engine and expect everything to be all right again. We didn't pour toxic chemicals over the roof or run them through the engine in the hope that we would fix the problem. In fact, occasionally, we would try that by buying some snake oil mixture, but even if by some miracle these potions worked for a while, the problem always came back because the underlying problem wasn't really fixed.

So, in the future, what we do now to cure cancer will look just as crude and ineffective as the "snake oil" treatments on my car. In probably ten years, scientists will be able to selectively turn off, or turn on, certain critical genes that control the growth of cells. When that day comes, a patient who is diagnosed with cancer will have a small sample of the tumor removed for genetic analysis.

In the laboratory, technicians will compare the genetic blueprint of the patient's cancer cells with his normal cells. The specific change that has occurred in the cancer cells will be identified. There may even be more than one change. No matter. The lab will be able to lay out for the doctor all of the relevant cellular changes for his cancer patient. The doctor will then select the exact medicine that will alter the patient's cancer gene profile and elect to change the cells back to normal by turning some particular gene off, or by turning on a particular gene sequence that will destroy the cancer cells.

The point here is that the cancer patient will be entirely free of his cancer without all the debilitating effects of current anticancer drugs. At this point in the near future, cancer will be a completely curable disease, and the war on cancer will be won.

We are on the brink.

CHAPTER 2

▼

WHAT BIOTECHNOLOGY MEANS FOR CANCER TREATMENT

The very thing that makes cancer cells so difficult to fight, their DNA, is also the cells' Achilles' heel. If we knew enough about how the cancer cells worked, how they were altered, we could stop them selectively, leaving the normal cells untouched. After all, this is what the body does successfully most of the time. This is where the human genome comes in. Knowing the blueprint in detail could help us to turn off the right switch in the cancer cells.

There are 24 human chromosomes containing 3 billion units of DNA. Each of us has 30,000 genes. The genome is the hereditary information in each of us. Just as your genes and your environment affect your personality, they affect the way cancer influences you, too.

Isolating a gene is a beginning. We can use the gene the way a detective uses a fingerprint (or now DNA), to search among the millions of molecules inside the cell for a protein product that matches the sequence of the cancer gene. When we know the location of the protein we can discover other proteins that frequent this chemical pathway, explore how these proteins interact to relay signals to the cell nucleus, and determine how a breakdown in signaling along this pathway contributes to disrupting the cell cycle. The focus is on seeing the precise molecular causes of cancer.

If a number of our genes become altered over time, they may begin producing abnormal proteins that cannot perform their assigned jobs in the cell. Let's say a gene has the job to relay growth signals to the interior of the cell, a critical process to the well-being of the cell. But with abnormal proteins, messages may never reach their destination. It is like a series of letters that gets lost in the mail. Without chemical guidance, a cell may begin to act blindly on its own—the first step in the multistep process that leads to acquired, or sporadic, cancer.

Characterizing the most frequent combinations of gene mutations that turn a normal cell into a tumor cell is one of the great challenges of genetics. Such information will have a profound effect in accurately diagnosing and treating the disease.

When scientists first began isolating inherited genes, it was hoped that these genes would lead to simple diagnostic tests that would tell people whether they would one day develop the cancers that run in their families. However, the story has turned out to be vastly more complex. Cancer susceptibility genes carry not one common alteration but rather hundreds of potential mutations, making the calculation of risk extremely variable. Moreover, family members sometimes have the same mutation in a cancer gene, and yet one sibling develops cancer and the other does not, suggesting factors that compensate for the altered gene and modify one's inherited risk.

While dramatic progress has been made in identifying the "major" cancer susceptibility genes, it is likely that genetic susceptibility in the population at large will be related to individual differences in subtle gene changes. These subtle gene changes may influence how people are affected by exposure to various environmental or hormonal factors.

Cancer is a genetic disease in which many factors, including diet, smoking, chemicals, sunlight, and viruses, are thought to cause alterations or mutations in our genes. An alteration can result in a change of the DNA material within a gene, or in excessive copies of a gene. Some alterations are inherited; others are acquired throughout life. When enough mutations accumulate, the normal processes inside the cell go awry, and tumors begin to grow.

Two gene classes play major roles in triggering cancer:

- Proto-oncogenes encourage cell growth.
- Tumor suppressor genes act as brakes on cell growth.

More than 100 cancer genes, each with its own blueprint for making a specific protein product, have already been identified— about 80 oncogenes and 20 tumor suppressor genes. (When normal proto-oncogenes are altered they are called oncogenes.) Mutations in proto-oncogenes produce too many growth-stimulating proteins or overly active forms of them. Mutations in tumor suppressor genes produce an inactive protein that deprives the cell of those crucial brakes needed to prevent inappropriate growth.

Because we know the normal functions of many of these cancer genes, we are able to speculate how these altered genes contribute to cancer development. In addition to the 100 cancer genes already known, however, there are more genes not yet discovered, and most cancers involve mutations of several genes.

Each person's cancer is distinct from another person's because each cancer is defined by its particular molecular pattern of altered genes. The more we learn about the molecular signature of a particular tumor or cancer, the easier it will be for doctors to make correct diagnoses, offer the best therapy, and accurately predict the outcome.

Most known cancer genes are involved in controlling cell growth, some are involved in DNA repair, and some in functions we don't yet know. For example, we now believe the two breast cancer genes, BRCA1 and BRCA2, are responsible for nearly all cases of familial ovarian cancer and approximately half of all cases of familial breast cancer. Genes implicated in colon cancer have also been identified. Here are some of the genes we know about:

- HER2/neu or ERBB-2 is a gene that when mutated has been detected in breast, salivary gland, and ovarian cancers.

- The SIS oncogene is a mutant or altered form associated with gliomas, a type of brain cancer.
- RET proto-oncogenes when mutant are associated with thyroid cancer.
- RAS proto-oncogene mutations have been detected in lung, ovarian, colon, and pancreatic cancers.
- APC (adenomatous polyposis coli) tumor suppressor gene mutations are found in almost all colon tumors and a large percentage of benign colon polyps.
- MSH2 and MLH1 when mutated are associated with a hereditary form of colon cancer.
- NF1 is a tumor suppressor gene that when altered is involved in cancers of the peripheral nervous system.
- The altered protein of the gene that suppresses p53 is associated with many cancers.
- NTS1/p16 is a tumor suppressor gene that when mutated is associated with both malignant melanoma and pancreatic cancer.

HELPING THE BODY HEAL ITSELF

Until recently cancer treatment had been designed to rid the body of cancer by cutting it out, poisoning it, or irradiating it. Now the focus is on finding ways to make the body itself combat the cancer rather than killing the cancer from the outside.

Research into various forms of immunotherapy and gene therapy to treat cancer has been going on for as long as 30 years. With the human genome solved and with data bank technology, we are on a faster track for putting these biotech therapies into practical use.

Some may be used along with existing chemotherapy or radiation. (Even traditional chemotherapy involves more than one drug to find the best results.) Now, with the emergence of the new biotechnologies, combination therapy will become more important. Doctors will be able to tailor combinations of therapies to fit particular patients depending on age, stage of disease, and particular molecular changes that caused the cancer.

Many of these drugs in early human testing may prove safe enough to take for years, perhaps for a lifetime. They may let us live in peaceful coexistence with cancer, transforming this dread disease into a chronic condition kept under control, the way diabetes is controlled with insulin.

DESIGNING DRUGS TO HIT THE RIGHT TARGET

There are many cancers, not just one disease. People often tell you that someone has "cancer," as if that word alone explained the person's condition. But it does not. Cancer is a group of many diseases. They are all different and are treated differently.

Cancer is not going to disappear as polio did almost immediately after the Salk and Sabin vaccines were made available. The most likely scenario is that cancer will be gradually transformed into a manageable chronic disease whose progress will be slowed or, in some cases, stopped. It will probably require a lifetime of medication to keep it under control. In many cases it will be similar to heart disease, where much progress has been made in reducing mortality.

We know the cause of cancer: the mutation of certain genes. Of the 40,000 human genes, only 300 to 400 are important for cancer. If those genes are not working, the cell either dies or becomes malignant. If a drug can knock out one or two of these target genes, the cancer can be stopped. We all accept that in time the treatment of cancer will be a lifetime routine. The more that you can strike at cancer itself, the less toxic and harmful the cancer treatment can be. We are embarking on a science-intensive form of cancer treatment. Now the scientific tools are there. We can design drugs that intervene at a specific place in the cancer process.

This "targeting" was discussed recently one evening on the *Charlie Rose Show* broadcast on public television. Rose gathered cancer specialists to talk about the recently approved Gleevec, a biotech drug that sends one particular form of leukemia into remission.

"We've achieved the blocking of some fundamental protein in the cancer cell," said Dr. Harold Vamus, president of Memorial Sloan-Kettering Cancer Center. "It's a major advance for the patient. For the scientist it is the fulfillment of the dream of finding that process." He told the audience that he believes "we know a lot of the targets. The question is, can we develop the molecules for those targets?" He also said he believes it is now possible to do the discovery at a much more rapid pace.

Dr. Vincent DiVita, director of the Yale Cancer Center, said, "Now we are getting sophisticated, every therapy is less morbid. This is proof of the principle [that molecular targeting is working]."

Dr. Paul Elder of the Dana-Farber Cancer Institute in Boston said his optimism was guarded. He mentioned tumor angiogenesis—blood vessels feeding tumors—as especially exciting. "If we can find a way to close all of the doors, then we can keep them closed." He added that the lack of toxicity was important. "We may be coming near the dawn of a new era. We will keep you alive longer so that you can benefit from the new targeted therapy."

This book serves as a guide to the new developments in cancer therapies. It sorts out for the reader some of the most interesting information for cancer therapies from the thousands of scientific papers and professional presentations that are available today. For example, Medline has over 34,000 citations for prostate cancer. The amount of information is a staggering mountain. This book helps you find the valuable nuggets in that mountain.

Dr. DiVita offered the best advice of all. "If your doctor tells you, 'There's nothing I can do for you,' don't believe it. There's almost always something we can do. You should take advantage of everything you can, because things are moving, and there's hope."

CHAPTER 3

▼

THE CANCER FRONTIER
Biotech Companies and the Emerging Therapies

Dr. Jonathan Lewis, M.D., Ph.D., the chief medical officer of the New York biotech company Antigenics, has an expensive gift pen on his desk high in the office towers of Rockefeller Center. On it, inscribed in gold, are the simple words, "You saved my life." They are the words of a grateful patient.

Dr. Lewis is a leader in the quest for a vaccine against cancer. At least five biotech companies are racing to find a workable vaccine against intractable diseases like pancreatic cancer, sarcomas, and kidney cancer. Dr. Garo Armen, chairman and CEO of Antigenics, says, "We must now think about reprogramming the immune system to fight cancer. After more than thirty years into the war against cancer, we see the death rates for solid tumors to be no better than they were years ago. This is because we have been taking the wrong approach to killing cancer cells."

Well, Antigenics is doing just that. It is trying to use the body's own formidable immune system to recognize and destroy cancer cells. It does this by using purified components of the cancer patient's own tumor cells to immunize the body against the individual's own cancer. Dr. Armen explains, "The body's immune system is very good at recognizing foreign proteins. That's why organ transplant patients must be carefully typed when they receive an organ from another person. But in cancer, the body's defense cells cannot recognize the cancer as a danger. Therefore, they do not mobilize against it."

Antigenics has been testing its vaccines at New York's Memorial Sloan-Kettering Cancer Center since 1997. The company uses the tumor tissue removed from cancer patients to extract special heat shock proteins, which carry peptides specific to the patient's own tumor. After purification, these proteins are injected back into the patient. After that the cancer patient's normal immune response takes over. The patient's special destroyer cells, called T cells, are alerted to the presence of dangerous proteins on cells circulating in the body. These T cells seek out and destroy any cells with those markers on their surface, a dead giveaway that they are cancer cells.

A cancer vaccine works in a way very similar to a smallpox or a polio vaccine. Harmless proteins from the disease-causing entity are introduced into the patient's skin, where immune cells recognize the foreign agent and mount an attack against it. While smallpox and polio vaccines work to stop viral infections before they start, cancer vaccines use the body's immune system to find tumor cells that are already present and are hiding from the body's defenses.

Once activated T cells find a tumor cell, they destroy it. Repeating the process over and over again, the immune system can gradually reduce the size of a tumor or eliminate it completely. Moreover, the T cells can reach hidden places in the body that no surgeon can see. They can go into the darkest recesses of organs and zap individual tumor cells that may wait for years before they grow into recognizable tumor masses. It's almost as if the vaccine gives the body a spring cleaning and gets rid of all cancer cells.

Antigenics developed a vaccine against kidney cancer at the University of Texas M. D. Anderson Cancer Center in Houston. After giving the special vaccine to 42 cancer patients, doctors saw that tumors in a number of patients had begun to shrink. One patient had a lump on his arm the size of an orange. Within weeks, the tumor had shrunk to the size of a pea. Doctors had advised that the man's condition was hopeless, but after seeing the results of the

Antigenics vaccine, they removed the remaining tumor. After more vaccine injections, this man remains free of his disease.

Another patient had moles removed repeatedly from many locations on his body. Pathologists diagnosed them as melanoma. After a recurring melanoma appeared in the man's liver in 1998, doctors advised against further surgery. They told his family that he would probably die within six months to a year.

After a relative found out about the treatment on the Internet, the man flew to M. D. Anderson. One of the hospital's leading surgeons operated in December 1998, but had to leave some tumor behind. The patient then received his first vaccine shots. After several months, the remaining tumor had not grown. It had stabilized.

In this melanoma group of patients who received their first vaccine therapies less than two years ago, 53 percent are cancer free or their cancer has stabilized.

Their physician, Dr. Omar Eton of M. D. Anderson, said, "We are very encouraged by the high percentage of disease-free patients in the trial so far."

Of 38 kidney cancer patients who received custom-made vaccines from Antigenics, 24 percent have been free of the disease or at least stabilized.

The company recently started two Phase II clinical trials testing its vaccine Oncophage for treatment of non-Hodgkin's lymphoma and sarcoma.

Antigenics' Dr. Armen said, "The recent advances in genomics point to the advantages of individualizing medicine to treat many of the major diseases. Antigenics is at the forefront of individualized medicine. Our technology platform has allowed us to develop therapeutics based on the individual antigenic fingerprint of diseased cells."

Dr. Lewis is always mindful of his role as a physician and surgeon. He knows from years of experience, many of them at Memorial Sloan-Kettering, that a vital part of treating cancer patients is to be sensitive to their needs as human beings. So much of the success of cancer treatments depends on the caring and love that's given to the patient by his family and his physician. To that end Antigenics has a psychologist on board to advise the company on the emotional needs of cancer patients. Dr. Lewis says, "We're trying so hard to do it right."

Antigenics is one of 300 biotech companies actively involved in genetic research, more than 100 specifically targeting cancer. This massive push is not because of a warm and fuzzy feeling about ridding humanity of this killer. The men and women who run these companies are in charge of spending millions of dollars of other people's money in research. They are hardheaded when it comes to betting their company's fortunes on research ideas, and they are collectively spending billions of dollars to find new and effective therapies for cancer because the science tells them it's possible.

Here are some of the ways they are working.

FIGHTING CANCER LIKE THE COMMON COLD: IMMUNOTHERAPY

The human body is well equipped to recognize and destroy foreign cells. Just look at what happens when you get a cold. Your body sees the virus particles as foreign and knows that they must be swept from the system. It immediately swings into action. The white cells in your blood find and attack the virus particles. Your temperature rises to make the environment unsuitable for the virus to survive. Fluids are mobilized to wash out the virus particles. When this all happens, we do not think that our bodies are mounting an immune response to the cold bugs. We just think we're miserable with a cold. But in truth, your body is putting up a very effective defense against this foreign organism. If it didn't we would all die of the common cold.

But in cancer, the offending cells are not outside invaders. They are our own cells. They have grown for years, selectively evading the body's defenses. Cancer kills us because in the end the cancer cells cannot be stopped by our body's immune response. But what if we could arrange things so that the body's natural immune defense could recognize and kill cancer cells? This would be perfect. The course of the disease would be much like a cold. First the body would see the cancer cells. Then it would mobilize antibodies to attack and kill the cancer cells. And finally, all the cancer cells would be swept out of our body, completely, never to return.

Targeting With Rifle Bullets: Monoclonal Antibodies

Monoclonal antibodies, commonly called MABs, are very much like the antibodies in our blood that fight bacteria and other foreign organisms. Nature has given us a fine array of these vital molecules. Without them we would die of overwhelming infections within days. But unfortunately they don't work against cancer cells.

We've known about monoclonal antibodies since 1970, and now scientists have discovered a way to make special antibodies such as Herceptin, which is so effective in treating some forms of advanced breast cancer (see Chapter 6) and other forms of the disease. These are very much like a rifle bullet compared to the shotgun approach that the natural antibodies in our bodies take. These rifle bullets can be directed against the cancer cells. The trick is to make the antibodies in such a way that they seek out the unique characteristics on the surface of the cancer cell, and leave all the other, normal cells alone.

The technique for producing MABs was developed in 1975 by Dr. Cesar Milstein and Dr. George Kohler at the Laboratory of Molecular Biology in Cambridge, England. Their accomplishment won them the Nobel Prize for Medicine in 1984.

MABs are created by injecting human cancer cells into mice and then removing the mouse cells that make antibodies against the human cancer. These cells are fused to immortal cells—cells that have lost their natural ability to die off. Combining the two cells results in tiny biological factories called hybridomas that endlessly produce a specific monoclonal antibody. Currently, scientists are exploring three major categories of monoclonal antibody therapy for use as high-tech weapons against cancer:

- **Unconjugated** antibodies seek out their target protein on the cell surface and attach to it. This binding itself kills the cancer cell, either by setting off a chain reaction of immune system events that destroys the cell or by making it unable to function.

- **Drug-conjugated** MABs are linked to a potent, cell-killing drug. This approach is called antibody-targeted chemotherapy. The drug kills the cell either by damaging its DNA or by inhibiting its function. Antibody-targeted chemotherapy sounds simple, but in reality its success depends on just the right combination of target antigen and MAB and their effective interaction. The first antibody linked to a chemical toxin is Mylotarg, approved by the FDA in May 2000 for the treatment of acute leukemia in certain patients 60 and older.
- **Radioisotope-conjugated** MABs are linked to radioisotopes. In binding with a tumor cell, the MAB delivers a dose of radiation directly to the cell that ultimately causes its death.

On Christmas Eve in 1989, an airline pilot, let's call him John Smith, went to the emergency room for a pulled abdominal muscle—or so he thought. It turned out to be a non-Hodgkin's lymphoma, an incurable cancer. His doctor told him it was probably his last Christmas. Mr. Smith went through the chemotherapy regimen, which made him quite sick but put the cancer into remission for several years. When it returned in 1997, he decided to try an experimental drug known as Zevalin, a monoclonal antibody attached to radioactive isotopes that act like guided missiles to deliver the antibodies to the tumors and kill the cancer cells. That treatment seemed to get rid of the cancer again. And three and a half years later, that pilot is still alive, having seen many Christmases since his first doctor's dour prediction. Zevalin was expecting approval in 2001, according to its maker, IDEC Pharmaceuticals. It is competing with Bexxar, made by Coulter Pharmaceutical, to become the first approved antibody with a radioactive warhead.

MAB therapy was almost abandoned in 1990 by the drug industry because it was so difficult to harness. It was often compared to "lightning in the body." But now that monoclonal antibody research is 25 years old, many of the barriers have been removed. This therapy doesn't cure everybody, and it has some side effects, but it is being used more, according to Samuel D. Waskal, M.D., president and CEO of ImClone Systems, a New York company developing these antibodies. He said this therapy has gone through a cycle of birth, death, and rebirth.

There were nine approved monoclonal antibody drugs in October 2000, up from only two in 1998. These include Genentech's Herceptin for breast cancer, Genentech and IDEC Pharmaceuticals' Rituxan for lymphoma.

There are more than 70 MABs now in clinical trials, half of them for cancer, according to Pharmaceutical Research and Manufacturers of America. They represent about 20 percent of all biotech drug trials.

To treat cancer, the aim is to kill cells. But some of the antibodies merely slow down the cells. In most cases, some doctors say, antibodies don't appear any more effective than chemotherapy in inducing remissions, though they have fewer side effects. So the best results might come along with other treatments. For some patients, however, antibodies have made quite a difference, as Mr. Smith can attest.

Because MABs are protein, stomach acid destroys them, therefore they must be given by injection or intravenous infusion. Large quantities are needed for treatment, and they cost about $10,000 a year.

Smart Bombs: Cancer Vaccines

Cancer vaccines are not meant to be preventative like smallpox vaccine or the Salk vaccine for polio. Your immune system can develop acquired immunity to a disease once it has been exposed to the disease because some cells, once activated, become memory cells. The next time the same antigen gets into your body, your immune system remembers how to destroy it.

However, a vaccine for cancer is designed to stimulate your body's immune system to fight cancer effectively, by using your own "killed" cancer cells. Cancer vaccine contains cancer cells, parts of cells, or chemically pure antigens and causes an increased immune response against the cancer cells already in your body. Cancer vaccines can be combined with additional cells or substances called adjuvants, which are known to boost the immune response.

Using T cells, obtained from the patient's own blood, scientists hope to destroy tumor cells selectively while leaving normal cells unharmed. The T cells are genetically programmed outside of the body to recognize and bind to tags, which are on many types of cancer cells. Then they are put back in the patient by intravenous infusion into the bloodstream. Since the normal action of a T cell is to destroy anything to which it binds, the altered T cells should go right to the cancer cells and kill them immediately. The biotech company in Seattle called Dendreon is a leader in this field.

There are several types of vaccines being studied with a total of 30 in production. They include the following:

• **Tumor cell vaccines.** Tumor cell vaccines use cancer cells from a patient in treatment (autologous vaccine) or from another patient (allogeneic vaccine). The cancer cells are killed, usually by radiation, before they are injected into the patient so they cannot form more tumors. However, the antigens on the tumor cell surfaces are still there and can stimulate an immune response. Tumor cell vaccines are being studied for use against melanoma, ovarian cancer, prostate cancer, breast cancer, colorectal cancer, and lung cancer.

Genzyme Molecular Oncology, a Cambridge, Massachusetts, biotech company, has been working with Dr. Steven Rosenberg at the National Cancer Institute to deal with melanoma. The company has developed a melanoma tumor vaccine that uses the body's own white cells to fight the tumor. Fifty-four patients with late-stage metastatic disease were treated with this vaccine. Most of these patients showed clinically significant tumor regression after this treatment.

GVAX is a vaccine developed by Cell Genesys that stimulates an antitumor immune response that targets and destroys tumor cells which persist following surgery or radiation therapy. Clinical studies are being conducted at the Dana-Farber Cancer Institute in Boston, where patients with lung cancer or melanoma are receiving vaccine made from their own "killed" cancer cells.

A study is being conducted at Johns Hopkins University in Baltimore with patients believed to have recurring prostate cancer. This trial hopes to determine whether the therapeutic vaccine can protect them from the recurrence and extend their survival. Another study is being conducted at three sites against colon cancer that has spread to the liver.

• **Antigen vaccines.** Antigen vaccines stimulate the immune system by using individual antigens instead of whole tumor cells that contain thousands of antigens. Now that the genetic codes of many antigens have been discovered, we can use gene-splicing techniques to produce these antigens in the lab. Some antigens can be made synthetically. Some cause immune responses in people with certain cancers. Others cause immune reactions to more than one kind of cancer. Several antigens may be combined in a single vaccine to cause a response to more than one antigen that may be on the cancer cell. Antigen vaccines are being studied for melanoma, breast, colorectal, ovarian, and pancreatic cancers.

• **Anti-idiotype vaccines.** Anti-idiotype vaccines are cancer specific and are being studied for melanoma, lymphoma, and other cancers. They are most promising against lymphomas because lymphomas have antigen receptors not present on normal cells. Every B cell or plasma cell that produces antibodies produces only one type of antibody. Each of these unique antibodies is called an idiotype. Anti-idiotype antibodies can be mass-produced. When the anti-idiotype antibodies are injected into the body, the immune system produces antibodies capable of reacting to the antigen on the cancer cell that caused the immune system to produce the original antibodies against it. Thus, the anti-idiotype antibodies can be used as a cancer-specific vaccine.

• **Dendritic cell vaccines.** Dendritic cell vaccines are specialized antigen-presenting cells that help the immune system recognize cancer cells. Dendritic cells break the antigens on the surfaces of the cancer cells into smaller pieces. Then they present those antigen pieces to T cells, making it easier for the immune system to react to them. To make dendritic cell vaccines, some of your own dendritic cells are removed and mixed with immune cell stimulants to reproduce the dendritic cells rapidly. The cells are exposed to antigens from the surface of the cancer cells. The dendritic cells and antigens are then injected back into the patient. These "trained" dendritic cells are better able to assist the immune system in recognizing and destroying cancer cells that have the same type of antigen on their surfaces. Vaccines are in clinical trials for prostate, colorectal, lung, and other cancers as well as melanoma.

• **DNA vaccines.** When antigens are first injected into the body as a vaccine, they produce the desired immune response. Over time, they are less effective because antibodies rapidly attach to them and they are destroyed. Bits of DNA can be injected into the body that instruct your cells to continually produce certain antigens. The altered cell produces the antigen on an ongoing basis to keep the immune response strong.

Tapping the Cell Phone: Cytokines

A new approach to advanced ovarian cancer involves special molecules called cytokines, immune system hormones. These are substances that the body's cells use to communicate with each other. It's a little like placing a tap on the cancer cell's telephone and then using the messages it sends to destroy it. A Phase I study of human interleukin-2, a type of cytokine, using genetically modified tumor cells in patients with metastatic ovarian cancer is being conducted at Duke University Medical Center.

Cytokines are called biological response modifiers (BRMs) because they can alter the interaction between the body's natural defense mechanisms and the cancer, thus improving the body's ability to fight the disease. Some BRMs occur naturally in the body, but others that imitate or influence natural BRMs can be made in the lab.

• **Interferons.** Interferons are cytokines that occur naturally in the body and were the first BRMs produced in the lab. There are three major groups of interferons: alpha, beta, and gamma. Alpha is the interferon most often used in cancer therapy. Interferons can boost the body's immune response to cancer and may also act directly on the cancer cells by inhibiting their growth or promoting their development into cells with more normal behavior. Some interferons may stimulate B cells and T cells, thereby strengthening the cancer-fighting function of the immune system.

A type of interferon alpha was the first BRM approved by the Food and Drug Administration (FDA) for cancer. It is used to treat hair cell leukemia, Kaposi's sarcoma, and chronic myelogenous leukemia. Interferon-alpha may also be effective against others such as renal cell carcinoma and some non-Hodgkin's lymphomas.

• **Interleukins (ILs).** Interleukins, like interferons, are cytokines that occur naturally in the body and can be made in the lab. Many interleukins have been identified, but IL-2 is the one most studied for cancer treatment. It stimulates the growth and functions of many immune cells that can destroy cancer cells.

• **Lymphokine-activated killer (LAK) cell therapy.** Large numbers of active cancer-fighting T cells can be produced in the lab by treating a small number of the patient's T cells with interleukin-2 (IL-2). When returned to the patient's bloodstream, these LAK cells are more effective against cancer cells than cells not treated with the hormone. This therapy has been successful in shrinking tumors in animals but, so far, not in humans. LAK cell techniques are being tested against melanoma, brain tumors, and other cancers.

• **Tumor-infiltrating lymphocyte (TIL) vaccine with interleukin-2 (IL-2).** Immune system cells deep in tumor tissue are called tumor-infiltrating lymphocytes. These cells can be removed from tumor samples taken from a patient and treated with interleukin-2. When injected back into the patient, these cells can be active cancer fighters. Immunotherapies using TILs are being developed for melanoma, ovarian cancer, and other cancers.

• **Tumor necrosis factor (TNF).** TNF is another cytokine. As in the case of interferons and interleukins, TNF stimulates the immune system to fight cancer. TNF also damages the tumor cells and the blood vessels within the tumor, but we still don't know how this damage occurs. The dose needed to kill the cancer, however, is so high it is toxic.

• **Colony-stimulating factors (CSFs).** CSFs, also called hematopoietic growth factors, do not challenge tumors directly. Several

CSFs have been identified that affect bone marrow cells. Bone marrow is an important part of the immune system because it is the source of all blood cells. CSFs stimulate the bone marrow cells to divide and develop into white blood cells, platelets, and red blood cells. CSFs are of great benefit when combined with high-dose chemotherapy. While the cancer drugs damage the white blood cells and make you more susceptible to infection, the CSFs stimulate the white cell production. This makes it possible to use higher doses of chemotherapy.

STARVING TUMORS TO DEATH: ANGIOGENESIS INHIBITORS

Without a blood supply to give them oxygen, cancer cells would die as surely as any other cell in your body. So if the blood supply to the cancer cells could be shut off, they would melt away. This is just what's happening with a new group of therapeutic agents called angiogenesis inhibitors.

The rapid growth of blood vessels in the body is a normal process that occurs during pregnancy, menstruation, and wound healing. In each of these conditions, as cells divide and grow, new capillaries are formed to supply needed blood. There is another situation in which blood capillaries proliferate: during cancer cell growth. Powerful natural compounds called angiostatin and endostatin that switch off the capillary growth. This is the hottest new area of research to combat several tumor types including breast, brain, and lung cancers. It would work without the toxic side effects of most current cancer medication.

Scientists from EntreMed, in Rockville, Maryland, led by Dr. Judah Folkman, have been able to completely eradicate human tumors in mice using angiostatin and endostatin. Dr. Folkman and his colleagues at the Harvard Medical School and Children's Hospital in Boston have shown that tumors rely on blood vessel development in order to grow, and that natural proteins exist that dramatically inhibit tumors by interfering with that process.

It was Dr. Folkman's hypothesis that tumors must promote the production of some antiangiogenesis substance capable of stemming the flow of blood to other tumor sites. Attempting to prove the theory, one of his associates, Dr. Michael O'Reilly, a surgeon, found the first such molecule, a protein called angiostatin, after screening dozens of tumors in mice. Angiostatin is currently being tested in patients at Thomas Jefferson University in Philadelphia, but that study is too new to have produced results. Continuing his work in Folkman's lab, O'Reilly subsequently found endostatin.

In November 2000, EntreMed released results from three clinical trials on endostatin. Data from over 60 patients with 20 different tumor types and over 4,000 individual administrations of endostatin were promising, so the studies will continue.

In the initial tests on 61 people at three U.S. medical centers, tumors in several patients stopped growing and actually shrank in two cases. One patient with an aggressive pancreatic cancer was treated with endostatin at Dana-Farber/Partners Cancer Center in Boston and reported to have seen his tumors shrink significantly and remain stable a year later, when most other patients in his condition would have been dead.

Based on results in mice, Folkman believes that the most effective way to administer endostatin may be continuously, 24 hours a day and seven days a week, through a tiny portable pump that patients can wear on their belts. Such a continuous infusion trial, requiring patients to visit the hospital weekly instead of daily, got under way in December 2000 at Amsterdam's Free University Hospital and Boston's Dana-Farber Cancer Institute. Plans are to treat 15 patients with continuous endostatin for one month, followed by a month of subcutaneously administered endostatin.

The National Cancer Institute (NCI) and biotechnology and pharmaceutical companies are moving as fast as possible to make angiostatin available for clinical testing, and NCI is ensuring that adequate resources are available. There are at least 11 compounds now in clinical trials that may target angiogenesis. Used in combination with a common chemotherapy agent, angiogenesis inhibitors completely eradicated human breast tumor cells that were implanted in mice. The compound used, called THP-dox, has been licensed to ILEX Oncology for clinical trials.

If ongoing clinical trials are positive, the agents now in late-phase clinical trials could be approved by the Food and Drug Administration and become available for general use as cancer treatments. These include marimastat, a matrix metalloproteinase inhibitor, and thalidomide, a drug with multiple mechanisms that has shown some evidence of biologic activity in gliomas (brain tumors) and Kaposi's sarcoma.

A patient at M. D. Anderson Cancer Center, one of the three hospitals where endostatin is being tested, had a 60 percent shrinkage of a sarcoma on his jaw. An advanced melanoma in a second patient stopped spreading after endostatin began last November and has remained stable.

A Canadian company, Aeterna, is conducting trials of its angiogenesis inhibitor Neovastat. Phase III trials are under way in America and Europe to use the drug for renal cell carcinoma. Results are expected by the summer of 2002.

Several companies are developing squalamine. Phase II studies are under way for treatment of non–small cell lung cancer. It will be administered with each cycle of chemotherapy. Additional trials are being planned for ovarian cancer, pediatric neuroblastoma, and other solid tumors. Celgene Corporation and the NCI are working together to develop antiangiogenic drugs. Bristol-Myers and OxiGene are developing combretastatin or CA4P. Phase I clinical trials involve 80 patients in the United States and England.

If the angiostatin and endostatin compounds can be successfully developed for testing in humans, the sponsor of the drugs can work with the FDA to permit patients who are not participating in clinical trials to have access to drugs (such access is often called "compassionate use"). This allows patients to receive promising but not yet fully studied or approved cancer therapies when no other satisfactory options exist.

Angiogenesis inhibitors don't really have to make tumors smaller to save lives. They just have to stop them from growing. But this makes it difficult to know if you are hitting your target. It's not as though you could look at a CT scan and see that the tumor is smaller. Another puzzler is the size of the dose needed. Because the drugs are not toxic, it is impossible to know how much is too much or how much is enough.

One similarity between EntreMed's anticancer approach and Aphton's Gastrimmune (see Chapter 10), a vaccine, is that they both target signals from growth factors, to essentially "starve" cancer cells. These "starving" approaches are generating increasing interest among cancer researchers. The Aphton approach directly blocks the key growth factor gastrin. Thus, it prevents gastrointestinal cancers from undergoing cell division and metastasis. EntreMed's combination drug therapy is designed to block the receptor for a key growth factor, which signals blood vessels to grow into and throughout solid tumors. Thus, EntreMed drugs indirectly prevent cancer cell division.

In great demand on the scientific circuit, Dr. Folkman spends much of his time speaking at cancer conferences. He has told of a man who said, "I have cancer without disease." Folkman believes that most people have tiny cancers lurking inside our bodies. The only reason they don't grow is that substances called antiangiogenesis factors keep new blood vessels from growing and feeding the cancer.

THE SMART DRUG STRATEGY: GENE THERAPY

In a 1999 horror movie the bad guys used gene therapy and genetic engineering to increase the size of a shark's brain. Naturally, like Frankenstein's monster, death and destruction soon followed when things got a little out of control. This is not what gene therapy is all about. The biotech companies using this new science to cure disease are the good guys, like David Nance, of Houston, whose company, Introgen Therapeutics, is developing a cure for lung cancer.

A gene can be delivered into the cells of a cancer patient with instructions to produce a specific protein inside the cell. It will be like delivering a time bomb to the cancer cell, set to go off at just the right time to destroy it. The ability to deliver a gene specifically to the tumor tissue, wherever it may be located within the patient, could allow treatment of metastatic disease, which is now unreachable by the usual techniques of radiation or surgery because we can't tell whether we got all the cells.

By 2030, scientists predict, every disease will have a treatment option based on gene therapy. This is a "smart drug" strategy that alters the patient's genetic blueprint and thus changes the course of a disease. Such custom-tailored drugs are on the horizon, and pharmaceutical and biotech companies are investing heavily in both of these approaches, which are certain to be treatment options, not only for cancer, but for many diseases.

Researchers from the M. D. Anderson Cancer Center have shown that gene therapy can in fact repair damaged genes and suppress tumors. The p53 gene, for example, the most common gene mutation found in cancer, puts the brakes on cell growth and forces cells to commit suicide if their DNA is damaged by sun exposure or smoking. P53 gene therapy is being tested on lung and prostate cancers and is now in clinical trials.

The adenovirus (common cold virus) combined with p53 was tested in almost 100 patients with head and neck cancer, and tumors shrank in almost 50 percent of patients. "There was very little toxicity, even with monthly injections," said Jack Roth, the thoracic surgeon who led the study. "It was a little surprising." P53 gene therapy is also being tested on lung and prostate cancers.

According to the National Institutes of Health (NIH), during the 1990s, more than 390 gene therapy studies were initiated, involving more than 4,000 patients and more than 12 medical institutions. Two-thirds of these tests were for cancer.

While the idea of gene therapy is simple—give healthy genes to people with defective ones in order to cure or treat a disease—delivering the genes is problematic. Delivery vehicles are called vectors; they direct genes into the proper cells and get them to function once they are there. Vectors are typically made by inserting genes into deactivated viruses that target certain cells, literally infecting them with healthy DNA.

Vical, a San Diego company, has preliminary results from 52 patients in a trial of 70 people to study gene therapy for advanced skin cancer. In that study, a gene that alerts the immune system to recognize and kill foreign tissue is administered directly into the tumors. Vical said 10 percent responded well with tumors shrinking about 50 percent or more. In another 15 percent of patients, the disease stopped progressing and tumor size was reduced.

CONFUSING ONCOGENES:
ANTISENSE THERAPY

When the rock group Talking Heads sang "Stop Making Sense," they weren't talking about DNA. But that's exactly what another experimental treatment is all about. This new antisense therapy seems to slow down cancer cells by confusing them. Antisense molecules are threads of nonsense DNA that block oncogenes by jamming their message and canceling the order for growth-promoting proteins.

Most diseases are caused by incorrect or excess production of proteins. Information required to produce these proteins is contained in genes in the DNA. To produce a protein, the cell first makes a messenger copy of the gene containing the information necessary to produce the protein. This messenger copy is called the mRNA. The message is then read by the cell and translated into the process to produce the protein. An antisense drug specifically binds to the mRNA to prevent the cell from making the target protein. Scientists use the information content of mRNA to rapidly design highly specific drugs. Because of their specificity, antisense drugs have the potential to be less toxic than traditional drugs. In addition, antisense drugs can be designed to treat not only cancer but a wide range of diseases including infectious, inflammatory, and cardiovascular diseases.

Currently, two antisense drugs are showing promising results:

• **Genasense.** In January 2001 scientists at Genta, Inc., reported that Genasense reduced levels of BCL2 protein, caused antitumor responses, and possibly extended the lives of the patients when it was used in combination with dacarbazine, a chemotherapy drug.

The company said the study involved 14 people with advanced melanoma and showed encouraging rates of durable response and survival. Antitumor responses were noted in 6 of the 14 patients, including a pathologically confirmed complete response in a 90-year-old woman with metastatic disease.

Genta's research platform is anchored in their antisense technology. Genasense, the company's lead compound, has received "fast track" and "orphan drug" designation from the FDA. The combination of Genasense plus dacarbazine is currently in a Phase III clinical trial in patients with advanced melanoma. If, as they believe, overexpression of the gene for BCL2 protein contributes to both inherent and acquired resistance to chemotherapy, radiation, and immunotherapy, then combined use of Genasense with these treatments should yield a marked improvement in outcome for patients.

• **MG98.** MG98 is another antisense compound, this one developed by MGI in Minnesota. In August 2000, they licensed the North American rights to MG98 and a complementary small molecule DNA methyltransferase (MeTase) inhibitor program. Both efforts are targeting cancers where tumor suppressor genes are silenced so they control the growth of tumor cells. Reactivation of the tumor suppressor genes is the goal of both efforts, with each using a different mechanism of action. MG98 has demonstrated anticancer activity in an ongoing Phase I dose escalation trial involving a variety of solid tumor types. Further development of MG98 is expected in certain solid tumors.

FORCING CELLS TO AGE NATURALLY: TELOMERASE

Research on an enzyme called telomerase isn't nearly as far along as antisense therapy, but investigators are excited about its role in controlling the life-and-death cycle of all cells, including cancer cells. All DNA strands are capped by telomeres, extra bits of DNA that snap off piece by piece every time a cell divides. Once the telomeres are gone, the cell stops dividing and grows old.

Telomeres are also thought to be the "clock" that regulates how many times an individual cell can divide. In contrast to tumor cells, which are immortal because they can divide forever, normal somatic human cells are mortal because they have a limited capacity to proliferate. New technology could reset the telomere clock.

The progressive shortening of telomeres may be halted in cancer cells by the presence of the enzyme telomerase. This enzyme maintains and stabilizes the telomeres, allowing cells to divide indefinitely. In almost all human tumors, telomerase activity is detected. It is hoped that a therapy can be developed that inhibits telomerase activity and interferes with the growth of many types of cancer.

Researchers at Geron Corp. in Menlo Park, California, and other firms are working on ways to block telomerase in cancer cells to force them to age and die like normal cells.

CHAPTER 4

▼

HOW CLINICAL TRIALS WORK FOR YOU

Cindy Margolis, a Richardson, Texas, mother of three young children, was diagnosed with incurable non-Hodgkin's lymphoma, which had spread cancer throughout her body. Her promising future would be cut short if she followed only the conventional radiation or therapy or bone marrow transplant. But Cindy was a physician who had inside knowledge about cutting-edge research and experimental treatment. She joined the clinical trial of a genetically engineered antibody, Rituxan, a drug that became the nation's first anticancer monoclonal antibody.

"Even though my type of lymphoma is still considered incurable, Rituxan has renewed my hope of raising my three children," Margolis said. Since then this drug that mobilizes the immune system against cancer has been approved by the Food and Drug Administration. (Read more about this drug in Chapter 11.)

Cindy is luckier than most cancer patients. Fewer than 3 percent of the 2 million adults who will get cancer this year know about clinical trials of the latest cancer therapy. In fact, one woman quoted in the press recently said, "I didn't even know what a clinical trial was." Compare that to the 25 percent of all AIDS patients who are being treated effectively with the latest drugs because they had a wealth of information about clinical trials. The same cannot be said for cancer.

When so few patients become part of the clinical trials, it impedes the search for cures. The National Cancer Policy Board, an independent advisory agency, found that although 8 million Americans require some form of cancer therapy, too many are not getting the best treatment. The cause: lack of good information on treatment options.

By nature, clinical trials are at the cutting edge of medicine. Tomorrow's standard treatments are found in today's trials. However, many people view clinical trials as the use of human guinea pigs in medical experimentation with more harm than good. The reality is that far more people are helped than hurt by American clinical trials.

The ideas for clinical trials often originate in the laboratory. Researchers develop a clinical protocol (the action plan) for a trial after laboratory studies indicate the promise of a new drug or procedure. Initial trials in people focus on feasibility and safety. As researchers gain further experience, later trials seek to determine whether the new approach benefits people and whether it has advantages over standard approaches currently in use.

Clinical trials are sponsored by organizations or individuals looking for better ways to improve health care. And in the United States these trials are subject to rigorous standards established by the government. It is the responsibility of the sponsor to see to it that a clinical trial is conducted in a scientifically sound and ethical manner in accordance with all laws and regulations. The National Cancer Institute (NCI) sponsors a large number of clinical trials in the areas of prevention, diagnosis and detection, and treatment.

The NCI Cooperative Clinical Trials Program knits together groups of academic investigators, cancer centers, and community physicians into an NCI-supported network of national scope. The network consists of a number of consortia (cooperative groups) that seek to define the key unanswered questions in cancer and then conduct high-quality clinical trials to answer them. This kind of cooperation makes it possible to have central administration and data collection for trials taking place at a large number of sites all over the country. The cooperative groups place approximately 20,000 new patients on clinical trials for cancer treatment each year. These are principally the large Phase III randomized trials that help establish the state of the art for cancer therapy. In addition, the groups coordinate and perform large trials in cancer prevention.

The Community Clinical Oncology Program (CCOP) makes clinical trials available in a large number of local communities by linking community physicians with researchers in cancer centers. Local hospitals throughout the country affiliate with a cancer center or a cooperative group. This means your doctor may be able to offer you a chance to participate in a clinical trial without your having to travel a long distance or leave your usual caregiver. Several of these programs also focus on encouraging minority populations to participate in trials.

THE THREE PHASES

Clinical trials in this country are divided into three phases. Once a drug or therapy has been comprehensively tested on animals, it can be administered to humans. This is Phase I. Because the drug is new and untested in humans, it is offered only to people who have no other reasonable options; that is, you have nothing to lose. If you go into a Phase I trial, you face the biggest risk because these drugs haven't been tested on humans before and their toxicity is not clearly understood. (Fewer than 5 percent of drugs ever get to the next trial phase.) Once the drug has passed the first phase and shows clear signs of being effective without undue risk, it is admitted to Phase II. This time it is offered to a broader group of patients to better establish its value as a new treatment. The final phase compares the new drug or therapy with existing treatments or no treatment at all. In Phase III, some people receive the new treatment, while others receive a more conventional treatment or a placebo (which only appears to be a treatment). However, if a treatment is clearly safer and more effective than the alternatives, the FDA will sometimes allow this part of the testing to be omitted. Thus, the treatment gets on the fast track to full FDA approval.

The National Cancer Institute lists 1,870 clinical trials that are open, or active, for the treatment of cancer.

According to the Pharmaceutical Research and Manufacturers of America (PhRMA), researchers are developing more than 400 new drugs to target cancer. Many of them, they say, are cutting-edge medicines that will be alternatives to standard radiation and chemotherapy treatments. The number of medicines now in the pipeline is nearly double that of six years ago. The research is being conducted by 170 pharmaceutical and biotechnology companies. The NCI is working in conjunction with some of the companies or by itself on 93 of the drugs. The medicines in development include 68 for lung cancer, 59 for breast cancer, 55 for colon cancer, 52 for skin cancer, and 52 for prostate cancer. The remaining ones are being developed for other cancers. According to PhRMA, 17 of the medicines have already completed 12 to 15 years of testing and are now in review.

Data from the Center for the Study of Drug Development at Tufts University indicate that out of thousands of compounds that are screened for drug development, only 250 enter preclinical testing, and 5 of those enter clinical testing. Only 1 of those 5 ever reaches the market.

When a clinical trial is completed, the researchers analyze the data and get the word out to the medical community and the public. In general, results are first reported in a peer-reviewed medical journal to bring the new approach to the attention of doctors and researchers, but this is really only a technicality. Trials reported in *The New England Journal of Medicine*, for example, are reported in major newspapers only one day after publication.

WHO PAYS FOR YOUR PARTICIPATION?

Do you know why there are more children with cancer in clinical trials than adults? Because the kids have advocates: their parents go to war with the establishment to make sure their children get the latest and best possible care. From 60 to 70 percent of children with cancer are enrolled in clinical trials, compared to fewer than 5 percent of adults. Such small numbers have hampered the search for cures.

Money is at the core of this problem. Until very recently, your health insurance was not likely to pay for your participation in a clinical trial. Such trials were classified as "experimental" and therefore not worth the risk to the insurance company. While drug companies might pay for the drugs, they did not always pay for the hospital care and lab tests that go along with participation in the trial.

Now some insurance companies will pay for some clinical trials, but there is no overall move to pay for any clinical trial—not yet, anyway. In 1999 in New Jersey, a coalition of medical insurers agreed to pay for experimental treatments in federal clinical trials. In other parts of the country, other insurers were beginning pilot programs to pay for valid studies.

Some drug makers offer the treatment free if you are willing to participate. But this depends on the type of trial. If a drug company is developing a new drug that they hope to get approval for, then they are more inclined to pay you for your participation. Other trials, such as those sanctioned by the NCI or other government agencies, are more likely to be covered by health insurers.

The fact that health insurance is beginning to pay is an important step. Previously, only in pediatric cancer did doctors, patients, and advocates work together to get children into clinical trials. The result is that now doctors can find out more quickly whether a treatment works. And this has contributed to the decline in death rates for children with cancer.

A WIDER WORLD OF INFORMATION

You have many things to consider before you join a clinical trial; balance the benefits and the losses. You get expert medical care, often free. On the other hand, you could be in a control group and not get the new drug therapy. There may be side effects to the treatment that could affect your lifestyle. In addition, participation may involve more time and medical tests than you would normally incur.

There is now a considerable amount of information on clinical trials on the Internet. Traditionally, the pharmaceutical companies recruited people with print, radio, and TV ads. Not everybody who comes through the Internet will be a perfect match, but it's a much quicker way to find the right match for a clinical trial.

If you visit each of the web sites you can find out where and when the trials take place, who is eligible to join, where they are conducted, and sometimes a list of questions to ask yourself and your doctor before you decide.

Since the end of 2000, several clinical trial sites have opened up on the web. At least four are up and running with more coming. Except for government sites, they are privately financed and geared to helping drug and biotech companies recruit people for their trials.

Some of the following web sites include clinical trials in all areas of medicine, so you have to search by geography, region, or type of cancer for the trials that will be suitable for you. Keep in mind that commercial sites on the web are not subject to government or peer review monitoring, so always check what you find with your doctor or other health-care professionals.

- **Cancernet.nci.nih.gov.** This is the National Cancer Institute's web site and lists all current clinical trials for cancer treatment, prevention, and diagnostic testing. You can also get information on clinical trials by calling the NCI's Cancer Information Service at 800-4-CANCER (800-422-6237).
- **Centerwatch.com.** This is the first private clinical trial site founded in 1996 as an outgrowth of a newsletter marketed to doctors and drug companies. A listing of trials categorized by disease is geared toward medical professionals. For more information, you can call their Patient Recruitment Office at 800-411-1222.
- **Emergingmed.com.** If you want to, you can provide your per-

sonal health information and this site will try to match you
up with a clinical trial. You will reveal your personal information only after a prescreening process.

- **Vertasmedicine.com.** This site is affiliated with doctors at
  Harvard and Tufts University and it plans to license its
  health information content to other sites. It also has a program for capturing medical data. This means you check a
  box to receive product information. You don't have to give
  your name to receive information. But the trade-off may well
  be worth it if it helps you get lifesaving treatment. This site
  and emergingmed match you to specific trials.
- **Acurian.com.** This site is a liaison between drug companies
  and patients. It has a link to Hopkins Health Views, from
  Johns Hopkins Medical Center. This site also gives you some
  useful tools, such as a list of questions to ask your doctors before you agree to participate in a clinical trial.
- **Hopelink.com.** This is a private software company managed
  by executives and others with health-care experience. You
  can locate a trial by the type of cancer, and this site, too, offers tools to enroll in an information network about the trials.
- **Americasdoctor.com.** This site appears to be more oriented
  toward health-care professionals.

In addition to these sites for general information about clinical
trials, you will find specific clinical trial sites in the following chapters in this book that detail information about particular cancers.
For example, Chapter 9, about lung cancer, includes comprehensive information about clinical trials for that cancer.

PART TWO

▼

WHERE TO GET
THE BEST AND LATEST
CANCER TREATMENT

CHAPTER 5

▼

WORKING WITH YOUR HEALTH-CARE TEAM

If the president were diagnosed with cancer, doctors and researchers would search for the latest information available on treatments that could save him. Top experts would be summoned to the White House. The president would be treated with the best and latest available. He would be given the best opportunity to defeat that cancer, to survive, and to return to good health.

For the rest of us, it's chancy. You may get the best care available or you may not. While teams of physicians and researchers would search the literature to make sure a president or a senator got the best there is, the same would not be done for you or me. Most of us assume that our doctor is up to date on the latest treatments. However, the facts are that this assumption is as naive as it is comfortable.

There is a very real chance that a potentially lifesaving treatment exists that your doctor does not know about. You simply don't know unless you have the latest information on your illness. That's where your health-care team comes in.

FIRST THINGS FIRST: YOUR ROLE ON THE TEAM

It may seem obvious, but it is very important to remember that you are the most important person on your health-care team. As with any type of health care you receive, you are a consumer of services, and you should not be afraid to ask questions about what you are getting and who is providing it.

You might consider these tips:

- When you go to meet with a doctor, nurse, or specialist, take someone else with you. It helps to have another person hear what is said and think of questions to ask.
- Write out your questions beforehand in order to make sure you don't forget to discuss any.
- Write down the answers you get, and make sure you understand what you are hearing.
- Don't be afraid to ask your questions or ask where you can find more information about what you are discussing. Being well informed is your most important task on the health-care team.

HIRING A DOCTOR

If you are diagnosed with cancer, seek out competent medical treatment right away, preferably from a board-certified specialist. But be aware of a few facts of life. First, you are responsible for the direction of your treatment. To put it in more familiar terms, you are the general contractor. It is you, or your family members, who must choose the right medical care. Just as you would hire an electrician to wire your house, you must contact and hire a physician to treat you for cancer. When you deal with an electrician, you don't expect to know what he knows about wiring. That's why he's the professional.

Normally, you would want to know something about the job at hand. If not the details of wiring, you would have an overall objec-

looking for one, ask your doctor, HMO, hospital, or social worker for a referral.

Home Health Aides: Extended Care

Another form of home care is from a home health aide. They are trained to assist people who are ill and need help moving around, bathing, cooking, or doing household chores. Some state Medicaid programs will pay for home health aide care, provided they are supervised by a nurse. However, private insurance or managed care plans rarely pay for a home health aide unless there is also a need for skilled nursing care. To find home health aide care, ask your doctor, nurse, or social worker. Remember to ask whether the charges vary according to income. Also, the National Association of Home Care (202-547-7424) publishes a free booklet, *How to Select a Home Care Agency*. The telephone yellow pages are another source, but be sure to check credentials. Find out whether the agency is bonded and ask for written references.

Rehabilitation Specialists: Help for Recovery

Rehabilitation services help people recover from physical changes caused by cancer or cancer treatment. They include the services of physical therapists, occupational therapists, counselors, speech therapists, and other professionals who help you physically recover from cancer. For example, physical therapy can help you rebuild the muscles in your arm and shoulder if you have had chest surgery.

Most physicians will refer you to rehabilitation if you need them. Be sure to ask if you think you might want them. Also, check to see whether these types of services are covered under your insurance plan. This varies according to the insurer. Additionally, some cancer or social service organizations may provide you with free rehab services if you are not insured for them.

Dietary or Nutritional Services: To Combat the Effects of Treatment

Cancer and cancer treatment can cause people to lose weight. For this reason, dietary or nutritional counseling and services are commonly prescribed for cancer patients. A dietician can suggest ways to get enough calories, vitamins, and protein to help you feel better and control your weight and can give you tips about increasing your appetite if you experience nausea, heartburn, or fatigue from your illness or treatment.

Most hospitals have registered dieticians on staff, and you can ask your doctor about meeting with them. If you are trying to locate a dietician in your community, be sure to ask about experience and training. Remember to check whether the services of a dietician are covered under your insurance. If not, ask your doctor, nurse, or social worker about community-based programs that offer free services.

Clergy: Spiritual Support Is Important

Prayer and spiritual counseling can be very important in coping with a serious illness such as cancer. Many people find it useful to get help from clergy or other spiritual leaders. There is no question that a strong sense of spirituality can help people face difficult challenges with courage and a sense of hope. Some studies show that people with cancer have less anxiety and depression, even less pain, when they feel spiritually connected. Even if your beliefs are challenged by your illness, don't be afraid to reach out to others for help. It is important to remember that you are not alone at this time.

Hospice Care: Help With Terminal Illness

Hospice care focuses on the special needs of people who have terminal cancer. Sometimes called palliative care, this type of care centers on providing comfort, controlling physical symptoms like pain, and giving emotional and spiritual support. Hospice care is usually provided at home, although there are hospice centers that operate much like hospitals and provide full-time care. Your doctor or social worker can refer you for hospice care.

Home hospice care is usually coordinated through a nurse, who then sends a home health aide, social workers, occupational therapist, clergy, or the type of specialist that is appropriate for the needs of the hospice patient. Hospice care is not for everyone. It is important to discuss this option carefully and get guidance from your doctor, nurse, or social worker.

PUTTING THE TEAM TOGETHER: FIND HELP AND HOPE

A diagnosis of cancer may be the most difficult challenge you or your loved ones will ever face. That is why it is important to find help and try to maintain your sense of hope no matter what your situation. Your team of health-care professionals is knowledgeable about the many different aspects of cancer: medical, physical, emotional, social, and spiritual. They are available to you as much or as little as you need, but it is difficult for them to know you need help unless you ask for it. Don't be afraid, embarrassed, or hesitant to ask questions. Voice your opinion, and seek the care you feel you need and deserve.

FINDING INFORMATION ABOUT TREATMENT

Information about cancer treatment is available from CancerFax, a fax-back document delivery service that makes some information from Physician's Data Query (PDQ) available via fax. PDQ is the NCI's comprehensive cancer database. To use CancerFax, dial 301-402-5874 and listen to the recorded instructions. Cancer information from PDQ also is available by sending an Internet e-mail message to cancernet@icic.nci.nih.gov with the word "help" in the body of the message; a contents list and instructions will be returned via e-mail.

You can contact PDQ Search Service by calling 800-345-3300 or sending a fax to 800-380-1575 (313-831-8929 outside the United States) or by sending an e-mail to pdqsearch@icic.nci.nih.gov.

CHAPTER 6

▼

BREAKTHROUGH TREATMENTS FOR BREAST CANCER

During the last decade of the 20th century, when women began demanding more research and better treatment for breast cancer, medical care began improving, even though the basic treatment remained surgery, chemotherapy, and radiation. Much of this gain has been achieved because conventional care has gradually improved over the years, the emphasis on earlier detection is bringing in breast cancer patients early enough to be treated successfully, and now new therapies emerging from a scientific understanding of the way cancer cells work.

The five-year survival rate for localized female breast cancer has risen from 72 percent in the 1940s to 98 percent today. There are now about 173,000 breast cancer cases diagnosed in the United States each year. There were about 43,700 deaths for this disease in 2000. Prostate cancer for men and breast cancer for women have the highest incidences for cancer in the United States. Female breast cancer ranks third in the number of new cases worldwide at 796,000 new cases, but fifth as a cause of death because of its relatively favorable prognosis. A few men also get breast cancer: about 1,300 a year. In the United States 43,000 women died of breast cancer in one year compared to 400 men.

The good news is that the earlier the treatment the better the survival. Naturally, the highest chance of cure is when the cancer has not spread outside the breast. Even if it has spread outside the breast, but in the same region, the survival is about 75 percent. That number decreases to 20 percent with distant metastases. But this is beginning to change with the widespread use of tamoxifen, Herceptin, Taxol, and other new therapies. There are 63 new drugs now under development for breast cancer. This is more than for any other type of cancer, according to a survey by the Pharmaceutical Research and Manufacturers of America.

GENETICS OF BREAST CANCER

No one knows exactly what causes breast cancer, but certain genes are linked to some types of breast cancer. The BRCA1 and BRCA2 genes were identified in 1997; fewer than 1 in 20 women with breast cancer carry these genes, but those who do often get the disease at a younger age. Between 5 and 10 percent of breast cancer cases can be blamed on an inherited tendency.

Women descended from European Jews have a higher-than-normal risk of getting breast cancer. Women in North America and Northern Europe have the highest rates of breast cancer; this variation may be due to diet. White women are more likely to develop breast cancer than black women, but black women are more likely to die from it. Asian and Hispanic women have a lower risk of developing breast cancer.

Another gene has been traced to breast cancer—HER2/neu—in 30 percent of women. In a healthy cell, the gene produces a protein that helps signal cells to grow normally and multiply. In women who have too much HER2, the breast cells reproduce out of control and spread through the body. A HER2 antibody, Herceptin® was developed by Genentech and has lengthened remission time for metastatic breast cancer.

MONOCLONAL ANTIBODIES

Lynn, 58, was diagnosed with breast cancer and the outlook wasn't good. The disease had spread to her lymph nodes, and even after chemotherapy and radiation, there were still signs of cancer in her bones and other parts of her body. "At first, I just wanted to go home and die," she said. "But then as the months passed, I began to realize that I wasn't the only one this had happened to. I realized it was up to me to fight this thing. No one else could do it for me."

Lynn refused to accept the death sentence and fought her way into clinical tests of the new treatment called Herceptin. She found that this new drug was easier to tolerate because unlike the other drugs she had taken, it had few side effects. The new treatment seemed to work. The signs of cancer in her vertebrae and pelvis had receded. After almost a year on the new treatment, Lynn had new hope for survival.

For the 30 percent of women whose tumors are fueled by the HER2 receptor, Herceptin offers a chance at living a little longer after the cancer has spread through the body, the scientific advisers concluded. "It's very exciting," said Dennis Slamon, M.D., of the University of California, Los Angeles, Jonsson Comprehensive Cancer Center, whose genetic research led to Herceptin. HER2-(human epidermal growth factor receptor 2) positive metastatic breast cancer is a fast-growing and deadly form of the disease offering approximately half the life expectancy of HER2-negative breast cancer.

Herceptin is the first treatment that specifically targets this aggressive form of breast cancer. It was developed to target a specific protein defect that contributes to the malignant progression of cancer. Routine tumor marker testing in women with breast cancer is critical for identifying those who are HER2 positive and who potentially would benefit from treatment with Herceptin.

Genentech genetically engineered an antibody that blocks excess HER2 to inhibit tumor growth and possibly even kill cancer. It's not a magic bullet—it helped only half the women who tested it. But adding Herceptin to chemotherapy or Taxol doubled women's chances that tumors would shrink. In women who already had failed standard therapy, Herceptin alone cut in half tumors in 15 percent of women. Amazingly, a handful of women went into remission. They weren't cured—most later relapsed—but one is alive six years later and another three years later.

"This is the biggest difference I've ever seen in Stage IV disease," said Larry Norton, M.D., of Memorial Sloan-Kettering Cancer Center in New York, one of the principal investigators of the Phase III study. Researchers took pains to express caveats, stressing that the data so far are based on only 12 months of follow-up. Dr. Slamon, the chair of the randomized trial, noted that data on survival, in particular, were "too early to declare."

A second Herceptin study at Rush–Presbyterian–St. Luke's Medical Center in Chicago reported that the drug extended the lives of several patients when used as a single agent in women with metastatic disease that had failed one or two prior chemotherapy regimens.

In clinical trials, some women who took Herceptin showed a complete remission of breast cancer. One was a Los Angeles corporate attorney who was diagnosed with cancer in 1994, during the same week her sister died of the disease. She was treated at UCLA and heard Dr. Slamon speak of the encouraging results of the Phase I and II trials of Herceptin. In early 1997, she volunteered to be part of the Phase III trials and was one of the last patients accepted. At first she took Herceptin in combination with traditional chemotherapy. Then, after successive scans showed that her tumors kept shrinking, she began to take Herceptin alone. Since early 1998 her tumors have almost disappeared. She continues to receive weekly doses of Herceptin from her doctor, and she has had no side effects.

In 1992, Lucy had abnormal findings in her annual mammogram. The doctor said it looked like calcification and should be followed up in six months. But Lucy is not a six months kind of person. She sought a second opinion from a breast surgeon. After a thorough exam, another mammogram, ultrasound, and a biopsy, the "abnormality" turned out to be cancer. Lucy's mother had died of breast cancer and she assumed she was about to die, too. She had a lumpectomy and the cancer was removed. She had 25 radiation treatments but no chemotherapy. However, her doctor decided to follow up with a course of Herceptin.

Overall, the most common adverse reactions related to Herceptin were chills and fever, primarily with the first infusion, in 40 percent of women. None of the women suffered the usual chemotherapy side effects like hair loss, mouth sores, and low blood cell count levels. An increased risk of heart dysfunction occurred in some women receiving Herceptin and other chemotherapy, but in most cases, this side effect was managed with medication. Herceptin can cause malfunction of the heart muscle or blood vessels, especially the left ventricular vessel.

The drug was approved by the FDA in 1998. Herceptin is also known by the generic name trastuzumab. Approximately 164,000 women have metastatic breast cancer in the United States today, according to estimates by Genentech, and the approval of Herceptin may offer the breast cancer patients who have this genetic alteration of the HER2 gene a better chance for a longer remission and survival.

Herceptin is approved for use in women with HER2-positive metastatic breast cancer. It's approved as both a first-line treatment, in combination with Taxol, and as a second- and third-line treatment by itself. The genetic alteration in the HER2 gene produces an increased amount of the growth factor receptor protein on the tumor cell surface that can be inhibited with the administration of Herceptin in patients with HER2-positive disease. Routine tumor marker testing in women with breast cancer is critical for identification of patients who are HER2 positive and who potentially could benefit from treatment with Herceptin. Herceptin is marketed in the United States by Genentech and internationally by Roche.

Knowing that a breast cancer overexpresses HER2 can definitely influence treatment decisions, according to Larry Norton, M.D., chair of solid tumor oncology at Memorial Sloan-Kettering Cancer Center in New York. Previously, routine testing for HER2 overexpression was not important because the results would not change how the cancer was managed. Now we know that proper choice of therapy may depend on this knowledge, so testing has become essential.

Testing is done on tumor tissue and should be done at the time of diagnosis. If you have breast cancer and want your HER2 status checked, ask your physicians to test for it at the time of biopsy or surgery or using their stored tumor tissue.

If you have advanced breast cancer and are interested in entering HER2 trials, you and your doctors may call the NCI's Cancer Information Service (CIS) at 800-4-CANCER (800-422-6237). More information about Genentech's work with Herceptin and about the drug itself is available from the company at 650-225-5759.

In 2000, the European Union approved the drug and it is currently being administered in Japan, Australia, and Canada. In March 2001, Genentech announced the results of a landmark clinical trial. Women with one of the most aggressive forms of metastatic breast cancer showed a significant survival benefit when treated initially with Herceptin and chemotherapy compared to chemotherapy alone. The findings were published in the *New England Journal of Medicine.*

"Herceptin represents a turning point in the treatment of breast cancer. The study results demonstrate that this targeted biologic approach is an important new treatment modality for metastatic breast cancer," said Dr. Slamon. "These results confirm that Herceptin with chemotherapy used as a first-line therapy offers women with HER2-positive metastatic breast cancer their best chance at increasing survival."

"The exciting results of this prospective, randomized study demonstrate the value of clinical trials in translating important laboratory observations into actual therapies that extend and save lives," said Dr. Norton, the study's senior author.

"Publication of the final results of the pivotal trial in a peer-reviewed journal is an important milestone for Herceptin," said Susan D. Hellmann, M.D., M.P.H., Genentech's executive vice president for development and product operations and chief medical officer. "Herceptin is one of only a few therapies to demonstrate this type of survival benefit for metastatic breast cancer. These results further underscore the importance for women with breast cancer and their physicians of understanding the aggressive nature of HER2-driven disease."

The most serious adverse effect was cardiac dysfunction, which occurred more frequently when Herceptin was administered with the chemotherapy compared to the chemotherapy alone.

"Cardiac safety is important when considering the use of Herceptin," said Dr. Slamon. "However, given the extremely poor clinical prognosis of women with HER2-positive disease and the fact that it is essentially incurable with current regimens, the risk of cardiac dysfunction must be weighed against the potential significant clinical benefit of Herceptin therapy when used within indication."

Four Phase III randomized clinical trials evaluating Herceptin as adjuvant therapy in early-stage breast cancer currently are enrolling or planning to enroll more than 10,000 patients at 800 sites worldwide.

"The next step is to see if the beneficial effects of Herceptin are seen in patients newly diagnosed with breast cancer with abnormal amounts of HER2," said Dr. Norton. "This is a critical focus of ongoing and planned clinical trials."

VACCINES

Many medical scientists predict that vaccines will join surgery, chemotherapy, and radiation as a major form of cancer treatment. In March 2001, Biomira, a Canadian biotech company, enrolled 1,000 patients in a Phase III trial of their vaccine Theratope for metastatic breast cancer. The trial is designed to find out whether Theratope vaccine can induce the body to create an immune response against cancerous cells. Patients are randomly assigned to one of two groups. One is given the vaccine, and the other gets only the protein that stimulates the immune response.

Final analysis of data from the Theratope vaccine Phase III trial is expected to begin in mid-2003. However, Biomira has planned two interim analyses for the Theratope vaccine trial so they can potentially make the vaccine available sooner to patients who need it. The first analysis was expected at the end of 2001.

"This large-scale Phase III study is extremely rigorous, and enrolling the greater number of patients is a significant accomplishment," said Alex McPherson, M.D., Ph.D., president and CEO. Trials are ongoing at over 120 clinical sites in North America, Europe, Australia, and New Zealand.

The vaccine consists of a protein marker (an antigen) that is carried on the surfaces of breast cancer cells, along with another protein that stimulates a general immune response. This double-barreled approach is designed to overcome the ability of cancer cells to "hide" from the body's immune system and to help it recognize and mount a specific attack against the cancer antigen.

Such vaccines are being tested on advanced cancer, but one day they may be used to prevent the disease from occurring. Preliminary results are promising. Side effects are few: some pain and swelling at the injection site.

ANTISENSE THERAPY

Genasense, mentioned in Chapter 3, is an antisense drug from Genta that has received "fast track" designation from the FDA. Preliminary clinical studies show it may be effective alone, but it is clearly even more effective combined with chemotherapy. The current program is set up to test that idea.

In July 2000 immune-deficient mice were given human breast cancer and treated with Genasense either alone or with doxorubicin, a common chemotherapy drug. When used alone, both these agents showed only modest activity, but in combination they showed a high level of antitumor activity.

Genta's programs are testing the use of Genasense as a pretreatment to reduce BCL2 protein production and then to administer state-of-the-art cancer therapy. Genasense treatment reduced BCL2 protein by 97 percent in breast cancer cells, and combined use with doxorubicin yielded a highly synergistic anticancer effect.

Dr. Raymond P. Warrell, Jr., Genta's president and CEO, said,

"This study follows an emerging concept in the scientific community with respect to control of cancer cell death. This concept suggests that there are balanced 'pools' of proteins that regulate either the initiation or the prevention of cell death. In cancer, alterations in the balance of these pools may be critical factors."

The study was published in July 2000 in *Clinical Cancer Research,* an official journal of the American Association for Cancer Research.

CHEMOTHERAPY

When breast cancer has spread, surgery is usually followed by a course of chemotherapy with a combination of drugs, such as doxorubicin, cyclophosphamide, fluorouracil, epirubicin, and others. More recently chemotherapy is being used before surgery to shrink the tumor so surgery is less drastic. Conventional chemotherapy drugs are also being combined with some of the new biotech drugs, which seem to make it more effective.

Chemotherapy Before Surgery

While chemotherapy has been used for decades as an adjuvant therapy following surgery, using it before surgery is relatively new. Because of findings from a recent clinical trial, physicians are now using chemotherapy before surgery to shrink breast tumors in some women with Stage II or Stage III breast cancer. A smaller tumor means more breast tissue is conserved in the surgery that follows. This allows many women the benefit of a less radical, and often less disfiguring, treatment option. As a result, more women who might have had a mastectomy are now candidates for therapy with chemotherapy followed by a lumpectomy.

In a trial involving more than 1,500 breast cancer patients, researchers found that breast tumor size was significantly reduced in 80 percent of the women who received chemotherapy before surgery. The number of women with larger breast tumors who could undergo lumpectomy nearly doubled after chemotherapy.

Researchers found that a preoperative regimen of the drugs

doxorubicin and cyclophosphamide allows more lumpectomies to be performed. It also decreases the incidence of positive lymph nodes in women with locally advanced breast cancer. Overall, 12 percent more lumpectomies were performed in the preoperative group. However, in women with tumors measuring 5.1 cm (2 inches) or more, it was less effective.

Myocet

A new way to prevent conventional chemotherapy drugs from being so toxic in treatment for advanced breast cancer is to coat the drug with tiny droplets. Doxorubicin, for example, is an effective chemotherapy against breast cancer first used in the 1960s, but it can damage the muscles and blood vessels of the heart. This damage is called cardiotoxicity. Heart failure can be as high as 5 percent in those receiving the recommended dose. But a study at McGill University and Jewish General Hospital in Montreal shows that fewer women developed this condition if the pill was coated.

Approximately 300 women participated in a Phase III trial of the coated pills known as Myocet. Investigators say the liposome-encapsulated doxorubicin passes through the heart and lodges in other organs, such as the liver and the blood vessels that feed tumors. Then it slowly dissolves and allows the doxorubicin to fight the cancer. This means doctors can give doxorubicin for longer periods without as much risk of cardiotoxicity.

However, Myocet is not yet approved in that country or the United States. It is approved in Europe. The approval of Myocet in the European Union represents a significant step forward for those women who suffer from metastatic breast cancer and their families, said Charles A. Baker, chairman and CEO of the Liposome Company.

Taxol and Taxotere

Taxol (paclitaxel) and Taxotere (docetaxel) are compounds derived from the yew tree. Taxol is made from the bark, and Taxotere is made from the needles. The two drugs share a similar mechanism in treating cancer. While they are used primarily for ovarian cancer, Bristol-Myers Squibb has received FDA clearance of Taxol for treatment of breast cancer under certain circumstances, such as when the cancer has spread beyond the breast and a combination of other chemotherapy drugs is not effective. It is also used if breast cancer recurs within six months of receiving adjuvant chemotherapy. Two clinical trials have shown that under these circumstances, Taxol was beneficial in 59 percent of patients.

A nationwide study of Taxol involved more than 3,000 women—the largest adjuvant breast cancer study ever conducted. The study compared doxorubicin plus cyclophosphamide (AC) alone versus AC followed by Taxol in women with breast cancer that spread to the lymph nodes under the arm.

The study results demonstrate a significant survival advantage in the Taxol group with a reduction in the risk of relapse of 22 percent and a reduction of 26 percent in the relative risk of death. This is a major advance similar to that seen nearly 30 years ago when it was discovered that combination chemotherapy after surgery improved breast cancer survival compared to surgery alone.

Dr. Nacia Faure, medical director at Bristol-Myers Squibb, manufacturer of Taxol, said the study clearly demonstrates that Taxol improves survival in patients with early-stage breast cancer. She says her company remains committed to researching new applications and developing Taxol to its fullest potential.

Taxol is generally well tolerated. The most common side effects are a lowered white blood cell count, hair loss, numbness in hands and feet, muscle or joint pain, diarrhea, and nausea. A less frequent but serious side effect is severe hypersensitivity reaction. This creates shortness of breath, low blood pressure, and rash.

Taxotere has shown good results in breast cancer, as well as ovarian and non–small cell lung cancer. In 1995, the European Union allowed it to be marketed for people with locally advanced or metastatic cancer. It is approved for use in more than 20 countries including all 15 European Union countries.

There are now 35 clinical trials with more than 2,500 patients worldwide including the United States. Taxotere in Phase II clinical trials has the highest overall response rate ever reported—56 percent—as a single agent in the treatment of advanced breast cancer that resists commonly available treatments including anthracycline. More than half the women who failed other therapies responded to Taxotere.

Taxotere's side effects are mostly manageable. Hair loss, low white blood cell count, skin rash, fluid retention, hypersensitivity, nausea, and diarrhea were reported during the trials. Taxotere is administered intravenously for one hour every three weeks. This is more convenient than other therapies, reducing costly hospital stays and allowing patients to spend more time at home.

Taxol and Gemcitabine

A Phase I study of combined gemcitabine, a standard chemotherapy drug, and Taxol for patients with breast and ovarian cancer is also showing encouraging results. Researchers in Italy used fixed doses of gemcitabine administered on days 1 and 8, and Taxol on day 1 of a 21-day cycle in patients previously treated for metastatic breast or ovarian cancer.

The trials included 45 patients, 31 with breast cancer and 14 with ovarian cancer. All were treated at seven different dose levels. Among 30 evaluated patients with metastatic breast cancer, there was a complete response in 4 and partial response in 12. The median duration of response was 31 weeks. One complete response and 5 partial responses were observed in 13 patients with ovarian cancer having a median response duration of 32 weeks.

Taxotere and Herceptin

Research suggests that combining Taxotere and Herceptin has more power in treating cancer than either drug used alone. Exisulind and CP461 are potential treatments for breast cancers that did not respond to Herceptin or Taxotere alone.

Cell Pathways is developing Apotsyn (exisulind) in combination with other systemic therapies for advanced breast cancer. A Phase I trial of Apotsyn in combination with weekly Taxotere was conducted. Full doses of each agent were given to patients.

Exisulind (Apotsyn) and CP461 are the first members of a new class of potential therapeutic agents called selective apoptotic antineoplastic drugs, or SAANDs, which have been discovered under the development by Cell Pathways. They selectively induce apoptosis, or programmed cell death, in abnormally growing precancerous and cancerous cells.

ANTIESTROGEN THERAPIES

Hormonal therapy has a systemic effect similar to that of chemotherapy. To fight breast cancer, drugs that block estrogen are used. These are targeted hormonal drugs, but are in no way similar to hormone replacement therapy. In fact, they do just the opposite. The most well known is tamoxifen, but several others are now becoming more widely used.

Tamoxifen

Tamoxifen was the first estrogen receptor modulator to be tested clinically. In the early 1990s, tamoxifen was still a cutting-edge treatment, but it is now standard practice. It is an antiestrogen used as a follow-up after radiation and surgery to prevent the growth of cancer cells that may have been undetectable at surgery. Subsequent clinical experience has demonstrated a remarkable risk-to-benefit ratio for tamoxifen.

Over a period of 15 years, 55 randomized trials involving over 37,000 women have been conducted. A study of all these trials showed that taking tamoxifen for 5 years substantially reduces recurrence of breast cancer and improves 10-year survival for all women regardless of age, menopausal status, or prior chemotherapy treatment.

In postmenopausal women, tamoxifen is used to prevent the cancer from recurring. Tamoxifen is not as toxic as most cancer-fighting drugs, but it increases the risk of endometrial cancer and deep vein thrombosis. For all women, including those whose tumors are estrogen-receptor negative, tamoxifen significantly reduces the risk of cancer in the other breast. Women who take tamoxifen for the recommended 5 years of therapy have the greatest reduction in the incidence of new primary cancer in the opposite breast.

It is estimated that 1 in 6 women could be prevented from relapsing, and 1 in 12 from dying, if the drug were given to all breast cancer patients after surgery. The study also found that young, premenopausal women, not just older women, benefited substantially from tamoxifen therapy, even for those whose breast cancer had spread to the local lymph glands. It also found that tamoxifen reduced the incidence of new cancers in the opposite breast by nearly half.

Breast cancer is an unusual disease because it can come back 10 or 15 years later. The new findings show that a lot of these late recurrences can be prevented by adjuvant treatment with radiotherapy, chemotherapy, and, in particular, the hormone treatment tamoxifen.

"This is the first time we've had good evidence on the effects of treatment on 15-year survival," said Sir Richard Peto, professor of medical statistics at the University of Oxford, U.K. He told the 2nd European Breast Cancer Conference, in September 2000, "These results, from a worldwide overview of 300 randomised trials, that included around 200,000 patients, are a lot better than we expected. It seems that we can at last talk about real cure," he said.

"The best evidence on the extent to which better treatment is saving lives is from the U.K., where tamoxifen was widely used from the 1980s, and where deaths from breast cancer in middle-aged women have fallen by 30 percent over the past decade. It seems as though several other European countries are now beginning to follow in the same direction."

Raloxifene also blocks the effect of estrogen on breast tissue and breast cancer. It is currently being evaluated to see if it can reduce a woman's risk of developing breast cancer. It is not recommended for women who already have breast cancer.

Toremifene (Fareston) is an antiestrogen drug similar to ta-moxifen. It is used for postmenopausal women with breast cancer that has metastasized.

In a study of estrogen-dependent cancer, black cohosh extract was administered along with the cancer drug tamoxifen. The herb appeared to work synergistically with the cancer drug to help block the proliferation of breast cancer cells: the combined effect was greater than the sum of the effects of each substance alone.

A New Use for Tamoxifen

In July 2000, the FDA approved tamoxifen to reduce the risk of invasive breast cancer in women with ductal carcinoma in situ (DCIS) following breast surgery and radiation. Tamoxifen is the first medication to be approved for DCIS, which accounts for nearly 20 percent of all newly diagnosed breast cancer cases.

Using tamoxifen to reduce the risk of invasive breast cancer in women with DCIS is an important advance. DCIS is a noninvasive breast cancer involving only the cells lining the milk ducts in the breast, with no evidence that the disease has spread outside of these ducts. Until the 1980s, DCIS was treated by mastectomy. Today, options also include lumpectomy, or lumpectomy plus radiation therapy.

"The effectiveness of tamoxifen has now been proven across all stages of the breast cancer continuum from risk reduction in women at high risk to the treatment of advanced breast cancer," said Jerry P. Lewis, M.D., senior director, clinical research, oncology of AstraZeneca, makers of tamoxifen, which they call Nolvadex.

The FDA submission was based on data from a study of 1,804 women with DCIS who had a lumpectomy and radiation therapy. Half of those patients were prescribed tamoxifen and half received a placebo. After an average follow-up period of more than five years, the researchers found that the addition of tamoxifen to the treatment regimen significantly reduced the incidence of invasive breast cancer by 43 percent.

The risk of endometrial cancer and blood clots in the lung and legs increases approximately two to three times for women taking tamoxifen. Stroke, cataracts, and cataract surgery also occur more frequently. More common side effects are vaginal discharge and hot flashes.

Arimidex

In 2000 the FDA approved Arimidex (anastrozole) as a new treatment option for postmenopausal women first diagnosed with advanced or locally advanced breast cancer whose cancers are hormone receptive.

Even though menopause greatly reduces estrogen production, hormones are still produced in the body in other places, such as the adrenal glands. In fact, an enzyme called aromatase circulates in many parts of the body and converts other chemicals into estrogens. In order to curtail this type of estrogen production, aromatase inhibitors have been developed. Arimidex is the first aromatase inhibitor to be approved for first-line treatment in the United States. Previously, it was approved only for use after tamoxifen treatment. Two pivotal studies found that Arimidex was as effective and as well tolerated as tamoxifen when prescribed at the time of diagnosis for women with advanced breast cancer.

The North American trial showed Arimidex had a statistically significant advantage over tamoxifen for time to tumor progression with an average of 11.1 months for Arimidex versus 5.6 months for tamoxifen. The European trial showed Arimidex was as effective as tamoxifen with respect to both time to progression and tumor response rate. Patients with estrogen-receptor-positive breast cancer received the greatest benefit from Arimidex.

Arimidex was first approved in 1996 as a treatment for postmenopausal women with advanced breast cancer whose cancer has progressed following treatment with tamoxifen. Arimidex is a nonsteroidal aromatase inhibitor that lowers the amount of circulating estrogens in the body. Arimidex and tamoxifen work in very different ways. Arimidex stops the production of estrogen from the adrenal glands (near the kidneys), a main source of estrogen for postmenopausal women. Tamoxifen interferes with the cancer cells' ability to use estrogen for fuel to divide and grow. Arimidex is also currently being evaluated in comparison to tamoxifen as an adjuvant therapy for early breast cancer in a multinational trial called ATAC (Arimidex, tamoxifen, and combination therapy) with results expected in 2001.

Letrozole

Research reports in 2001 indicate letrozole (Femara), another aromatase inhibitor, is also better than tamoxifen as a first-line therapy for postmenopausal women with advanced breast cancer. Researchers from 18 nations designed a comparative Phase III study to compare how effective and well tolerated it is compared with tamoxifen as first-line therapy.

Participants included 907 patients who had estrogen-receptor- and/or progesterone-receptor-positive breast tumors or in whom both receptors were unknown. They were divided into two groups and randomly assigned a once-a-day dose of letrozole or tamoxifen.

The letrozole reduced the time of progression of the disease by 30 percent—regardless of the dominant site of disease, receptor status, or previous antiestrogen therapy.

Aromasin

Aromasin, a hormone inactivator, is currently indicated for the treatment of advanced breast cancer in postmenopausal women whose tumors have stopped responding to antiestrogen therapy such as tamoxifen. It may also turn out to be a preventative. It is the first in a new class of oral hormonal inactivator therapies being studied for the first-line adjuvant (after surgery) and neoadjuvant (before surgery) treatment of breast cancer. Aromasin (exemestane tablets) may limit the growth of an existing tumor and prevent cancer development in high-risk patients.

Aromasin is an aromatase *inactivator* that prevents the aromatase enzyme from producing estrogen, which some breast cancer tumors need for growth. This contrasts with aromatase *inhibitors*, which only interfere with the aromatase enzyme in a reversible manner.

Early results from a Phase II study comparing Aromasin with tamoxifen in advanced breast cancer show an improved response rate. This means Aromasin slows the tumor growth. Women treated with Aromasin also experienced fewer side effects (fatigue, pain, hot flashes, sweating, and nausea) compared to those treated with tamoxifen. Based on these promising preliminary clinical data, the European Organization for Research and Treatment of Cancer (EORTC) expanded this study to a Phase III trial.

In the neoadjuvant treatment approach, Aromasin is provided to patients in an effort to shrink large primary breast cancers prior to surgical removal. This method of treatment is important for women who are considering breast-conserving surgical options rather than a mastectomy. In a sample of 13 postmenopausal women with estrogen-receptor-positive breast cancer, Aromasin provided over the course of three months resulted in a median tumor volume reduction of 83 percent (as assessed by ultrasound).

Zoladex

ZEBRA is the name of the largest study ever to compare hormonal therapy with standard chemotherapy. The study involved 1,640 pre- and perimenopausal women with early breast cancer.

Results from the ZEBRA (Zoladex in Early Breast Cancer Research Association Trial) study show that treatment with Zoladex (goserelin) is as effective as standard chemotherapy for pre- and perimenopausal women with hormone-sensitive, node-positive early breast cancer. For these women, chemotherapy is currently the accepted standard treatment approach following initial surgery. However, the large doses of standard chemotherapy produce some harrowing side effects like hair loss, severe nausea and vomiting, and the risk of life-threatening infection.

In the hormone-sensitive group of patients (73 percent), Zoladex was shown to be equivalent to standard chemotherapy in terms of disease-free survival. In addition, Zoladex was not associated with the distressing and debilitating side effects routinely observed with chemotherapy.

The ZEBRA study was set up to find out whether these benefits would also be seen in the treatment of early breast cancer, and to find out whether Zoladex would prove to be as effective as chemotherapy for these young women.

RADIATION THERAPY

In the past, breast conservation treatment (BCT) meant a lumpectomy followed by six weeks of external radiation. This is the equivalent of a mastectomy in terms of survival rates. While BCT has strong emotional appeal for women who want to save their breast, the six-week cycle of radiation has been a deterrent in the past. This is especially true for women who live or work far from the facility and have to stay either in the hospital or nearby for the time.

Brachytherapy is internal radiation therapy that places a radioactive substance directly into the breast tissue next to the cancer. It has been called a "smart bomb" because a powerful radiation source is temporarily inserted into the cancer site so that, using computerized technology, oncologists can treat only the tumor and spare healthy surrounding tissues. The NIH is sponsoring a new study of radiation treatment that tracks women with early-stage breast cancer and their treatment with high dose rate (HDR) brachytherapy, an outpatient radiation therapy.

Cancer was found in both breasts of Rita, a 25-year-old woman who had watched her aunt, singer Minnie Riperton, lose a battle with breast cancer at 31. Fortunately, Rita's cancer had not yet spread to her lymph nodes.

Rita received the innovative brachytherapy that reduced the radiation cycle from six weeks to five days. This was the first study of HDR brachytherapy to focus on Stage I and II breast cancer at hospitals throughout the United States and Canada.

Rita is now 38 and a 13-year survivor. "When you're sick, people don't know what to say to you. 'Oh, poor Rita, she's so young.' I could see them looking at me with pity, which I didn't want because it made me feel like I was going to die." Rita now works with the American Cancer Society on the annual Minnie Riperton Run and Family Walk.

Data suggests that approximately 71,000 women a year would be eligible for this protocol. A study by the National Institutes of Health excluded women who may have an increased risk of microscopic disease in multiple areas of the breast.

Radiation for BRCA1 and BRCA2 Mutations

To answer concerns of patients and physicians, researchers in the United States and Canada examined whether radiation therapy could be safely delivered to women with early-stage breast cancer and BRCA1 or BRCA2 genetic mutations. They found that it can. Some women with these genetic mutations reject radiation therapy in favor of mastectomy because radiation is known to cause DNA damage. The presence of a BRCA1 or BRCA2 breast cancer susceptibility gene would result in a greater sensitivity to injury from radiation. However, according to lead investigator Lori Pierce, M.D., a radiation oncologist at the University of Michigan School of Medicine, the study shows that radiation is both safe and effective for treating early-stage breast cancer.

The study compared 71 women with BRCA1 or BRCA2 mutations to 213 women with sporadic (nonhereditary) breast cancer. Women in both groups had Stage I or II breast cancer and all received BCT. Five years after treatment, the researchers found no differences between the two groups in side effects after radiotherapy or in survival and the rate of cancer recurrence in the treated breast.

Radiation therapy helps prevent cancer recurrence in early-stage breast cancer regardless of whether a woman has a BRCA1 or BRCA2 mutation, according to current research. But as researchers expected, women with the mutations were almost 20 percent more likely to eventually develop cancer in their unaffected breast. They should discuss with their doctors ways to treat the existing cancer as well as prevent cancer in the opposite breast.

Radiotherapy Booster

A major international trial has produced the first firm evidence that giving extra radiotherapy to patients with early breast cancer substantially reduces the risk of recurrence. The results were so clear-cut that medical scientists believe that clinical practice should be changed immediately, particularly for younger women.

The findings are from the 5,569-patient multicenter study carried out by the European Organization for Research and Treatment of Cancer (EORTC). The study included 32 institutions from nine countries. The aim of the study was to see whether a booster radiation dose would reduce the risk of local recurrence of the tumor in women who had undergone breast-conserving surgery. The majority of patients (95.5 percent) had undergone complete removal of their tumor. All the patients had radiation to the whole breast. Some received a boost localized to the tumor bed area, while the control group received no further radiotherapy.

After a median follow-up of over five years, only 109 patients in the booster group had suffered a recurrence compared with 182 in the control group—a reduction in risk to date of nearly 50 percent. The largest benefit was seen in women aged under 40, where the chances of recurrence were cut by 54 percent. Patients will be followed up for many years to see whether booster doses will also cut mortality.

LASER TREATMENT

Photodynamic Therapy

Research at the University of Buffalo (UB) offered new hope of effective therapy for breast cancer lesions deep in the chest wall. Photodynamic therapy (PDT) has shown promise in lung and other cancers. However, it may have much wider application than previously thought.

Thomas S. Mang, Ph.D., has found that by manipulating the amount of a light-sensitive drug and the intensity of the laser beam that activates it, he can successfully treat cancer cells deeply embedded in the chest wall without damaging surrounding normal tissue. This low-dose PDT approach has resulted in complete healing in nearly 90 percent of 102 recurrent breast cancer lesions.

PDT was developed at Roswell Park Cancer Institute, the site of UB's basic cancer research programs. It is thought to have significant potential for treating certain types of cancers. So far PDT has been approved in treating non–small cell lung cancer and obstructing esophageal tumors. It is being used on an experimental basis for several other tumor types.

Cancer cells have a propensity to absorb higher-than-normal concentrations of photosensitive drugs. When exposed to light from lasers, these drugs become toxic and destroy the malignant tissue. Since normal tissue surrounding tumors also absorbs a certain amount of the drug, the goal is to find a drug-to-light ratio for each tumor type in order to kill the most tumor cells while sparing the most normal tissue.

In the study involving breast cancer lesions that had formed on the chest wall, Dr. Mang lowered the standard dose of a photosensitive drug, Photofrin. The standard drug dose would not have allowed them to use enough light to reach deep enough to kill the tumor cells without destroying normal tissue. By lowering the drug dose, the small amount of the drug in normal tissue bleaches out before it does any damage, and by delivering more light, doctors can reach deeper into tumors where the drug concentration is still high enough to kill cancer cells.

Dr. Mang and Ronald R. Allison, M.D., UB associate professor of clinical radiation oncology, treated nine patients with a total of 102 chest wall lesions. All the women had undergone surgery, full-dose radiation, and multiagent chemotherapy. According to Dr. Mang, 89 percent of the lesions healed completely without scarring after PDT. Of the remaining lesions, 8 percent became smaller. Three percent of women did not respond to the treatment.

Microwave Therapy

Celsion Corporation of Columbia, Maryland, began Phase II clinical trials of its breast cancer treatment system in early 2001.

The company's investigational breast cancer treatment system is based on technology developed at Massachusetts Institute of Technology (MIT) for the Star Wars Initiative. It focuses microwaves directly on cancerous cells in order to kill them with targeted heat.

According to Dr. Augustine Cheung, Celsion chairman and chief scientific officer, the treatment will address two major groups of patients. Patients normally expected to undergo mastectomy will, after Celsion's treatment, be able to undergo a lumpectomy instead. "This is a far more conservative procedure that may enable the patient to preserve her breast," said Dr. Cheung. The second group is patients with smaller tumors who would be candidates for a lumpectomy. The Celsion system would ablate these smaller tumors completely.

Celsion Corporation is a research and development company developing medical treatment systems for cancer and other diseases using focused heat technology delivered by patented microwave technology. The company works with leading medical institutions such as Duke University Medical Center, MIT, Harbor UCLA Medical Center, the University of California at San Francisco, Montefiore Medical Center, Memorial Sloan-Kettering Cancer Center in New York, and Duke University.

New Laser Treatment

Improvements in breast imaging have made it possible for doctors to find and diagnose breast cancer at a very early stage. A new procedure being tested at Rush–Presbyterian–St. Luke's Medical Center in Chicago holds promise for eliminating the need for surgery in women with small breast cancers. This procedure uses a laser delivered through a needle to destroy tumors detected by mammography.

During this new procedure the patient lies face down on a special (stereotactic) X-ray table enabling the doctor to have precise visualization of the tumor. Under local anesthesia the laser needle is inserted into the tumor and the second needle (a thermometer) is placed next to it. Laser energy is then delivered through a thin fiber inside the laser needle until the temperature around the tumor reaches 140°F, at which point all cancer cells are destroyed. The entire procedure takes approximately one hour, and the patient is kept under observation for another hour before leaving the hospital.

These women must also have lumpectomy afterward to prove that the laser beam has killed all the cancer cells.

In preliminary trials using laser therapy, 40 patients with breast cancer have been treated with no complications other than minimal pain requiring Tylenol tablets. Laser therapy is not appropriate for women with large breast cancers or those that cannot be clearly seen on mammogram.

PREVENTION STRATEGIES

Mastectomy

Women with a high risk of getting breast cancer because they have the BRCA gene mutations have sometimes had prophylactic mastectomies so they cannot get breast cancer. This drastic measure has been the subject of controversy for years. But researchers at the Mayo Clinic believe it actually does protect them from getting the cancer.

A decision to proceed with prophylactic surgery is extremely complex and personal and should follow a thorough discussion about one's underlying cancer risk and all options for clinical management, according to Lynn Hartmann, M.D., professor of oncology at the Mayo Clinic in Rochester, Minnesota. She presented her findings at the 91st annual meeting of the American Association for Cancer Research in San Francisco in 2000. Mayo Clinic researchers have been tracking the health of women who have opted for prophylactic mastectomy because of a family history of breast cancer. From 1960 until 1993, 214 women underwent the surgery, Dr. Hartmann said. Of those, 3 women later developed breast cancer and 2 women died of the disease. Breast tissue covers a large area of the chest and it is nearly impossible to remove all breast tissue surgically. Even one cancer cell left behind can wreak havoc later.

Among the women in the study, 28 carried BRCA genes with known deleterious or suspicious mutations. None of these women developed breast cancer, Dr. Hartmann said, although one of the women did contract ovarian cancer.

Of women who test positive for BRCA, only about 10 percent are interested in prophylactic mastectomy. For the rest, she said, the treatment of choice has been close surveillance for signs of breast cancer with frequent mammography. Tamoxifen is also on the prevention table now.

Women with BRCA mutations who undergo prophylactic mastectomy reduce their risk of contracting breast cancer about 90 percent.

Tamoxifen

Serious doubt about healthy women taking tamoxifen to prevent breast cancer is raised by a nationwide study that indicates these women have a high risk of developing endometrial cancer. At the same time, scientists add, the survival benefits from tamoxifen among women with breast cancer far outweigh the risks of endometrial cancer.

Early results of the Breast Cancer Prevention Trial (BCPT) showed a 45 percent reduction in breast cancer incidence among tamoxifen users, but neither of the two European trials with tamoxifen confirmed the BCPT findings.

Long-term use of tamoxifen can create cancer in the lining of the uterus. Constant vigilance and periodic testing with ultrasound and other techniques will catch the cancer early enough to treat and cure it. This is why long-term users of tamoxifen need to report any vaginal bleeding. It could indicate uterine polyps, which, when excised, may be benign.

Maspin Testing

Preliminary findings suggest there may be a way to recognize whether breast cancer is likely to spread. This could be a key to recognizing and giving more intensive care to women whose breast cancer is more likely to relapse. This key may be a protein called maspin, which is produced by epithelial cells.

Dr. Pier Francesco Ferrucci of the European Institute of Oncology in Milan has been studying 48 women who have had surgery and aggressive chemotherapy to treat their high-risk breast cancer. In all the women, breast cancer cells were found in the bone marrow and blood.

The researchers measured a range of substances associated with breast cancer in the tissue and blood samples. These substances included cytokeratins (which confirm the presence of epithelial cells) and mammaglobin (which shows the presence of cells deriving from breast tissue) as well as the protein maspin. This protein has only recently been shown to have the ability to suppress tumors. While the exact mechanism is not yet known, it may inhibit the growth of new blood vessels needed to feed the cancer cells.

Dr. Ferrucci and his colleagues found that in general, women with higher levels of maspin were less likely to relapse. And the effect was particularly pronounced in ten of the women, who had 20 or more lymph nodes showing breast cancer. After around 15 months' observation, eight of these women had not relapsed, and all had high maspin levels. The two women in this group with low maspin levels had developed secondary cancers of the liver and lung.

So far, the study simply found an association between the amount of maspin produced by breast cells and reduced risk of relapse. However, the findings are backed up by similar results recently published on other tumors derived from epithelial cells. It's hoped this will lead to a test that could routinely help doctors identify some of the women more at risk of relapse. This will mean they can prescribe more appropriate care and treatment. More trials on bigger groups of patients still need to be done.

THE NEED FOR MORE CLINICAL TRIALS

Experts in the treatment of breast cancer seem to agree that most women with breast cancer that hasn't spread should take a combination of chemotherapy drugs for three to six months after surgery to make sure any remaining cancer cells in their bodies are killed. In addition, women whose breast cancer may have been stimulated by estrogen should undergo hormonal treatment with tamoxifen for five years after surgery regardless of age. Evidence also indicates that radiation therapy in addition to chemotherapy or hormonal therapy can benefit women at high risk of recurrence. Those include women with evidence of cancer in at least four lymph nodes or when the primary tumor is advanced.

A panel of cancer experts at an NIH-sponsored conference in 2000 stressed that Taxol and related drugs may be effective against cancer that has spread to other organs. But Taxol remains unproven for therapy following the surgical removal of a localized breast cancer.

However, the scientists emphasized the importance of clinical trials. According to Patricia Eifel, M.D., a radiation oncologist at M. D. Anderson Cancer Center in Houston, there's even more compelling evidence of the long-term advantage of adjuvant chemotherapy and tamoxifen. Several panel members emphasized that answers to important questions about adjuvant therapy hinge on clinical trials and that these trials need better support from doctors and more participation by patients. The panel said there was a "critical need" for clinical trials to evaluate adjuvant chemotherapy in women over age 70.

In fact, the older the woman, the less likely she is to receive a full range of treatment for breast cancer. Women over age 80 with early-stage breast cancer frequently do not get a full range of treatments, even after considering their health and treatment preferences, according to a study conducted by the Lombardi Cancer Center, Georgetown University Medical Center in Washington, D.C. The study, involving researchers at 29 hospitals across the country, was published in 2000 in the journal *Cancer.*

Specifically, women 80 years and older were less likely to be referred to a radiation oncologist, and after breast-conserving therapy, they were more than three times more likely not to receive radiation therapy. The risk of cancer recurrence approaches 40 percent within 10 years when radiation is not given after a lumpectomy, well within the life expectancy for most older women.

The study also found that older black women seem to be less likely than older white women to receive radiation after lumpectomy. Researchers note that while the sample of black women was fairly small, this finding of differences in breast cancer treatment patterns by race is consistent with other research.

WHERE TO FIND INFORMATION ABOUT BREAST CANCER

The National Alliance of Breast Cancer Organizations (NABCO)
9 East 37th Street
New York, NY 10016
Telephone: 888-80-NABCO
Web site: www.nabco.org

NABCO is the leading non-profit resource for information and education on breast cancer in the United States, and a national force in patient advocacy. The organization provides information to medical professionals and their organizations, patients and their families, and the media. NABCO also provides action alerts on pending clinical trials and works closely with the National Cancer Institute.

The National Breast Cancer Coalition (NBCC)
1707 L Street, NW
Washington, DC 20036
Telephone: 202-296-7477
Fax: 202-265-6854
Web site: www.natlbcc.org

This is a network of organizations and individuals involved in a grassroots advocacy effort in the fight against breast cancer. Its main mission is to eradicate breast cancer through action and advocacy.

Self-Help for Women with Breast or Ovarian Cancer (SHARE)
1501 Broadway
New York, NY 10036
Hotline: 866-891-2392
Telephone: 212-719-0364
Breast cancer information in English: 212-382-2111
Ovarian cancer information in English: 212-719-1204
Information in Spanish: 212-719-4454
Fax: 212-869-3431
Web site: www.sharecancersupport.com

This organization provides support and other services for all affected by breast and ovarian cancer. There are many events that bring people together and a monthy newsletter.

The Susan G. Komen Breast Cancer Foundation
5005 LBJ Freeway
Suite 250
Dallas, TX 75244
National breast cancer helpline: 800-I'M AWARE (462-9273)
Web site: www.breastcancerinfo.com

The foundation strives to eradicate breast cancer by advancing research, education, screening, and treatment.

Y-ME National Breast Cancer Organization
212 W. Van Buren
Suite 500
Chicago, IL 60607
Hotline in English: 800-221-2141
Hotline in Spanish: 800-986-9505
Telephone: 312-986-9505
Web site: www.y-me.org

This group provides information, support, and education for patients, families, and those touched by breast cancer.

ONGOING CLINICAL TRIALS FOR BREAST CANCER

There are literally hundreds of clinical trials in various stages of development around the world. To list them all here would be misleading because by the time you read this book, some trials may have closed and many others may have opened. Clinical trials have specific eligibility requirements that may eliminate many cancer patients. The few trials listed here are only a sampling of the trials that may be open to you. The best way to locate clinical trials appropriate for your situation is to ask your doctor, check the web sites listed in Chapter 4, and call the biotech companies listed in Appendix C.

1. A Phase I pilot study of p53 (264-272) peptide vaccine and tumor-specific mutant p53 peptide vaccine in HLA-A2.1 patients with Stage IV, recurrent, or progressive adenocarcinoma of the breast. The study will try to determine whether vaccination with these peptides can induce or boost the cellular immunity of these patients.

   Contact Malgorzata Wojtowicz of the Center for Cancer Research in Bethesda, MD, at 301-435-5371.

2. A Phase I study of yttrium Y90 monoclonal antibody B3 followed by stem cell transplantation in patients with relapsed or metastatic breast cancer. This will determine the maximum tolerated dose of this therapy. A total of 20 to 30 patients will be accrued for this study over two to three years.

   Contact Nicole McCarthy of the Center for Cancer Research in Bethesda at 301-496-4916.

3. A Phase I/II study of high-dose chemotherapy followed by stem cell transplantation and immunotherapy with activated T cells, interleukin-2, and sargramostim in patients with Stage IIIB or IV breast cancer. A total of 60 patients will be accrued for this study over three to four years.

   Contact Lawrence G. Lum of the Roger Williams Medical Center in Providence, RI, at 401-456-2672.

4. A Phase II trial of Herceptin plus interleukin-2 in patients

with metastatic breast cancer who have failed prior Herceptin therapy.

Contact Charles L. Shapiro of the Arthur G. James Cancer Hospital at Ohio State University in Columbus at 614-293-7530.

5. A Phase III randomized trial of first-line Herceptin alone followed by a combination of Herceptin and paclitaxel in women with HER2-overexpressing metastatic breast cancer. Approximately 170 to 250 women will be accrued for this study.

Contacts are in Italy or Switzerland. Chairing the study is Aron Goldhirsch at the Swiss Institute for Applied Cancer Research at 39-02-574-894-39.

CHAPTER 7

▼

BREAKTHROUGH TREATMENTS FOR OVARIAN CANCER

While ovarian cancer doesn't usually strike women until middle age—the average age is 61—there have been some high-profile cases in younger women such as the actress Gilda Radner and the editor Liz Tiberis, both of who wrote books about their experiences before they died.

Because early detection is difficult, the symptoms of ovarian cancer are rarely discovered until it is advanced. Lately, however, more effective chemotherapy has been developed with new drugs and biotech therapies like cytokines, vaccines, angiogenesis inhibitors, and photodynamic therapy. Several studies are also looking at the use of aspirin or the hormone progestin to prevent recurrence of the disease.

In 2000 there were about 23,000 new cases of ovarian cancer in the United States, according to the American Cancer Society. About 14,000 women died from the disease. If this cancer is caught early, the five-year survival rate is about 95 percent. But because there is no effective screening test, ovarian cancer is difficult to detect. About 25 percent of these cancers are diagnosed before they have spread beyond the ovaries.

While epithelial cancer is the most common type of ovarian cancer, two other types account for about 10 percent of the cancers.

The epithelial type begins with the surface cells of the ovary; it affects mostly middle-aged and older women. Younger women are vulnerable to the germ cell tumors that occur in the egg-producing cells. Another rare type is stromal tumors that occur in the tissue that holds the ovary together. This is the tissue that produces estrogen and progesterone. Stromal tumors can develop at any age.

Medical scientists believe that fewer than 10 percent of ovarian cancers can be blamed on a genetic predisposition to the disease. If a woman has a BRCA1 (breast cancer) gene mutation, she has a 40 to 60 percent increased risk for ovarian cancer over her lifetime. (For a discussion of BRCA gene mutation, see page 95.) There is no conclusive evidence of other risk factors.

A pelvic examination can detect an enlarged ovary and this may be associated with ovarian cancer. The CA125 blood test is also useful in detecting ovarian cancer. CA125 is a protein antigen that is found in high levels in the bloodstream of many cancer patients. The specificity of CA125 is rather low, however, so elevated levels can be caused by noncancerous conditions. Also, some women with ovarian cancer do not have elevated CA125. Some imaging techniques such as ultrasound, CT, and MRI allow a doctor to see any tumor that may be present in an ovary, so if the CA125 is suspicious, these tests can confirm a diagnosis. A laparotomy, in which a small incision is made to open the abdominal cavity and inspect the internal organs, is often needed to be sure. In addition, recent studies indicate that a blood substance called lysophosphatidic acid appears elevated in women with gynecological cancers. Another test being studied evaluates a soluble form of an epidermal growth factor receptor (EGFR) that appears lower in women with this cancer.

CONVENTIONAL TREATMENT

Treatment for ovarian cancer usually is surgery followed by chemotherapy. Sometimes radiation is used as well. If the cancer is diagnosed during a laparotomy, then the surgeon will remove the ovaries, uterus, fallopian tubes, nearby lymph glands, and nearby fatty tissue. In other words, as much cancer as possible will be removed from the abdomen. This must be done with extreme care so as not to rupture the tumor and let cells spill out and spread the cancer. The chemotherapy used after surgery is usually a combination of cisplatin and cyclophosphamide. More recently, cisplatin has been combined with Taxol, and this has improved survival. Other drugs used include etoposide and topotecan.

Epithelial ovarian cancer is generally responsive to chemotherapy, but the cells may grow again in the future. When that happens, additional cycles of chemotherapy are used. Sometimes a platinum compound with or without added taxane is given. Germ cell tumors are often treated with a chemotherapy combination known as BEP—bleomycin, etoposide, and cisplatin.

CHEMOTHERAPY

Taxol

Taxol has been used to treat cancer in hundreds of thousands of patients around the world and is currently used, alone or in combination, as a first-line treatment for ovarian cancer. It is also used as a second-line treatment for cancer that has metastasized. Taxol and Paraplatin combined are the drugs most commonly used as a first-line treatment of ovarian cancer.

In 2000, the FDA approved a novel, shorter administration regimen for Taxol injection for the treatment of advanced ovarian cancer. The drug is approved for a new dosing regimen based on results of a Phase III worldwide clinical trial.

The new regimen recognized the greater effectiveness of Taxol in combination with cisplatin in a three-hour regimen every three weeks, as compared to the standard therapy of cyclophosphamide followed by cisplatin. Taxol is also approved for use in advanced ovarian cancer over a 24-hour infusion period given in combination with cisplatin every three weeks. The new three-hour regimen offers women the advantage of being treated as an outpatient without the need to stay in the hospital.

The results from this study confirm that Taxol and cisplatin have a significant survival benefit compared to previous regimens, according to Renzo Canetta, vice president of clinical oncology research at Bristol-Myers Squibb, which makes the drug.

The trial enrolled 680 women with Stage IIB through IV ovarian cancer. They received either Taxol-cisplatin or cisplatin-cyclophosphamide. The women receiving Taxol showed improved overall survival, compared to the others. Also, the disease did not progress as quickly. This increased survival was greater no matter the age, stage of disease, or grade of disease. Subsequently the other women in the studied were given the Taxol regimen, too.

The study confirmed the safety of the three-hour Taxol infusion with cisplatin. The combination reduced the normal chemotherapy side effects like lowering the white blood cell count, anemia, nausea, and other common side effects. One possible side effect of the Taxol is a severe allergic reaction causing shortness of breath, low blood pressure, and a rash. This means women with severe allergies may not be able to take Taxol.

Irofulven

The interim Phase II clinical trial of irofulven, sponsored by the National Cancer Institute with MGI Pharma, tried to determine the response rate of treatment with irofulven in women with recurrent or persistent ovarian cancer. Participants in this trial already had had treatment with another drug or combination of drugs, or their tumors had reappeared within six months of treatment. Two of the patients could not be evaluated, but the remaining 15 showed these results:

- Five had a greater than 50 percent reduction in tumor mass lasting from five to nine cycles of therapy.
- Two had stable disease (less than 50 percent tumor shrinkage), one for two and the other for at least eight cycles of therapy.
- Four withdrew after one cycle of therapy because of sickness or fatigue.

- Four discontinued treatment after two or three cycles because the disease progressed.

Mild to modest nausea and vomiting, as well as decreases in white
blood cells or platelets, were reported as side effects.

In addition to this trial, laboratory results focused on irofulven's
mechanism of action and its use in combination with radiation or
other chemotherapy agents. Cell signaling pathways controlling
irofulven-induced cell death in different tumor cell types were
identified. Additional lab studies showed that irofulven may be
combined effectively with a number of standard antitumor treatments including gemcitabine, mitoxantrone, the active metabolite
of irinotecan, and gamma radiation for different tumor cell types.

Hexalen

An option for second-line treatment with Hexalen, a pill form
of chemotherapy, is also available now. In studies women responded to Hexalen when they did not respond to previous first-
line therapy. Hexalen (altretamine) is approved in the United
States and more than 20 other countries for persistent or recurring
ovarian cancer. In the multicenter trial by the Southwest Oncology
Group, two-year survival rate for 97 women was 75 percent. Side effects are mild compared to other chemotherapy.

According to Dr. David S. Alberts, associate dean for research at
the College of Medicine and Arizona Cancer Center at the
University of Arizona, Hexalen may be important in managing recurrent ovarian cancer.

EXPERIMENTAL TREATMENTS

Cytokines

A Phase I study of human interleukin-2 using genetically modified tumor cells in patients with metastatic ovarian cancer is being

conducted at Duke University Medical Center in Durham, North Carolina, by Drs. Andrew Berchuck and H. K. Lyerly. Interleukin-2 is a special molecule called a cytokine, a substance that the body cells use to communicate with each other.

Dr. Berchuck is a professor in the department of obstetrics and gynecology at Duke. He studies the molecular events that underlie the development of ovarian and endometrial cancers. He also provides clinical care to patients at Duke. He can be contacted at 919-684-3765.

Gene Therapy

Another promising approach is being tried in a trial at the National Institutes of Health in Bethesda, Maryland. Here women with advanced ovarian cancer are being treated with anti-CD3 stimulated peripheral blood lymphocytes. These cells have been treated with a gene that tells the white blood cells to seek out and kill the cancer cells in the body.

Vaccines

Avax Technologies announced in September 2000 that its vaccine OVAX had received "orphan drug" designation from the FDA, which gives the company the financial incentive to develop the drug. In two trials of OVAX, the therapy appeared to induce immune responses and possibly extended survival in women with advanced ovarian cancer. In the first trial in 1999, nine women were treated with seven weekly injections of OVAX after surgery and chemotherapy. Eight of the nine women were alive after more than two years, and three were relapse free. In another study, eight of ten women demonstrated positive immunological reaction.

OVAX is prepared from the woman's own tumor tissue taken at the time of surgery. It is administered following standard chemotherapy.

The Avax studies of advanced ovarian cancer patients were conducted by David Berd, M.D., professor of medicine, and Charles

Dunton, M.D., professor of obstetrics and gynecology, both of Thomas Jefferson University in Philadelphia. (The company's MVAX is currently sold in Australia for third-stage melanoma.)

Photodynamic Therapy

The University of Pennsylvania is the exclusive clinical trial site of a novel treatment that may help prevent ovarian cancer from recurring. A photosensitizing chemical and laser light combine to produce a reaction that destroys tumor cells. No one is quite sure why, but normal cells are usually spared during this photodynamic therapy. "As best we can tell, the drug goes into all cells throughout the body, but normal tissues seem to clear it very quickly, in a matter of a few hours. Tumor cells appear to retain it for several days," explained Eli Glatstein, M.D., clinical director of radiation oncology, who is co-investigator. "This window of time allows us to target the tumor cells."

After a Phase I trial while Glatstein was at the National Cancer Institute, some women appeared to be free of the disease after treatment even though they came to the trial with advanced cancer and were not expected to survive.

Now in Phase II trials led by Penn radiation oncologist and principal investigator Stephen Hahn, M.D., women participating receive Photofrin II, a photosensitizing chemical, as outpatients. They return in two days for an exploratory laparotomy to remove the tumor. If the tumor can't be removed, the laser light is used.

Recurrent ovarian cancer usually involves widespread cancer in the peritoneal area and the laser light needs to reach many sites. To accomplish this, the doctors infuse a saline solution mixed with a common nutritional substance, Intralipid, into the woman's abdomen. The Intralipid diffuses the light throughout the solution and gets into all the nooks and crannies to bathe the area with light of the appropriate wavelength. The women remain at the University of Pennsylvania Cancer Center for several days for follow-up care with their physicians.

The most common side effect is to make the skin supersensitive to sunlight for as long as ten weeks.

GENETICS OF OVARIAN CANCER

Women with a strong family history of ovarian cancer should ask their doctors about taking a test to see if they have a defective BRCA1 or BRCA2 gene. These genes—for breast cancer 1 and 2— are felt to be responsible for nearly all cases of familial ovarian cancer and approximately half of all cases of familial breast cancer. Most women have normal copies of one or both of the BRCA1 and BRCA2 genes, which produce a cancer-preventing substance. Some women have a genetic defect in one of their two BRCA1 genes, or BRCA2 genes and don't produce a normal amount of this cancer-fighting substance. These women are at very high risk of getting breast or ovarian cancer over the course of a lifetime.

You inherit one copy of each of your genes from your mother and a second copy of each of your genes from your father. (This is why you look about half like your mother, and half like your father.) If one of your parents has a defective BRCA1 gene or BRCA2 gene, there is a 50 percent chance you may inherit their defective copy, and a 50 percent chance you may inherit their normal copy. If you inherit a defective BRCA1 gene or BRCA2 gene, then each of your children has a 50 percent chance of inheriting it from you.

HEREDITARY VERSUS SPORADIC OVARIAN CANCER

Women with advanced BRCA hereditary ovarian cancer survive longer than women with sporadic ovarian cancer. Researchers at Memorial Sloan-Kettering Cancer Center in New York studied women with ovarian cancer to determine whether hereditary ovarian cancers had distinct pathological features compared to those that are not hereditary. Jewish women were studied because the BRCA 1 and 2 mutations are common in this ethnic group.

While the two types of cancer were found to have similar disease characteristics, researchers found the women with the inherited type were diagnosed earlier than the others. Hereditary cancers were rarely diagnosed before age 40 and were common after 60.

But the average age at diagnosis was 54 compared to 62 in the other groups. They studied women with the same grade and stage and initial treatment. The hereditary group remained disease free longer after chemotherapy compared to the other group. There was a 25 percent decrease in death for the hereditary cancers.

According to background information in the article, about 10 percent of all epithelial ovarian cancers are associated with the genetic mutation. The BRCA genes function as tumor suppressors.

WHERE TO FIND INFORMATION ABOUT OVARIAN CANCER

The Gilda Radner Familial Ovarian Cancer Registry
Roswell Park Cancer Institute
Buffalo, NY 14263
Telephone: 800-OVARIAN (5682-7426)
Web site: www.ovariancancer.com

This organization's help line for high-risk women is a telephone support service run by volunteers. Just call the 800 number and ask for a help line volunteer to contact you. Call if you have a question about familial ovarian cancer, or if you would like information on registering.

Self-Help for Women with Breast or Ovarian Cancer (SHARE)
1501 Broadway
New York, NY 10036
Hotline: 866-891-2392
Telephone: 212-719-0364
Breast cancer information in English: 212-382-2111
Ovarian cancer information in English: 212-719-1204
Information in Spanish: 212-719-4454
Fax: 212-869-3431
Web site: www.sharecancersupport.com

This organization provides support and other services for all affected by breast and ovarian cancer. There are many events that bring people together and a monthly newsletter.

ONGOING CLINICAL TRIALS FOR OVARIAN CANCER

There are literally hundreds of clinical trials in various stages of development around the world. To list them all here would be misleading because by the time you read this book, some trials may have closed and many others may have opened. Clinical trials have specific eligibility requirements that may eliminate many cancer patients. The few trials listed here are only a sampling of the trials that may be open to you. The best way to locate clinical trials appropriate for your situation is to ask your doctor, check the web sites listed in Chapter 4, and call the biotech companies listed in Appendix C.

1. AstraZeneca has a new platinum-based drug in development for women with ovarian cancer. It is interested in recruiting patients into clinical trials. This drug is designed for women with ovarian cancer that is resistant to the chemotherapy regimen of platinum plus Taxol. It is also meant for women whose cancer has recurred after this treatment. Patients must be 18 or older and must have been treated with chemotherapy regimens other than platinum and Taxol combinations.

   The trials are being conducted in several locations in the United States. To learn more about enrollment and locations near you, call 800-236-9933.
2. Geneara is conducting clinical trials for its anti-angiogenesis drug, squalamine, at several locations. In Denver, trials are being conducted at the University of Colorado Health Sciences Center and the Rocky Mountain Cancer Centers. Trials are also under way at the UCLA Clinical Research Unit

in Los Angeles, Vanderbilt University Medical Center in Nashville, St. Vincent's Hospital in New York, and Women and Infant's Hospital in Providence.

3. SuperGen in San Ramon, California, is conducting clinical trials of its drugs Camptogen and Rubitecan.

4. The National Cancer Institute is conducting clinical trials for HPV16E6 and E7 vaccines.

5. The interleukin-2 cytokine is being tested at Duke University Medical Center.

6. The OVAX vaccine is being tested at Thomas Jefferson University Medical Center in Philadelphia.

7. Genzyme Molecular Oncology and the National Institutes of Health in Bethesda are conducting clinical trials of HSP65.

8. Interleukin-12 is in trials sponsored by the National Cancer Institute and Genetics Institute.

9. The University of Pennsylvania is conducting trials of intraperitoneal photodynamic therapy to evaluate the effectiveness of photodynamic therapy in women with ovarian cancer (and also in patients with gastrointestinal cancer).

CHAPTER 8

▼

BREAKTHROUGH TREATMENTS FOR PROSTATE CANCER

High-profile prostate cancer survivors like New York Yankees manager Joe Torre and Michael Korda, editor in chief of Simon & Schuster, who wrote a book about his own experience called *Man to Man*, have raised the consciousness of many men about new choices for prostate cancer therapy.

The natural history of prostate cancer is poorly understood. It is primarily a disease of older men. Postmortem studies show that the vast majority of prostate cancers never develop into clinically apparent disease. It has been estimated that for a 50-year-old man with a life expectancy of 25 years, there is a 42 percent lifetime risk of having microscopic cancer, a 9.5 percent risk of having clinically evident cancer, and a 2.9 percent risk of dying of prostate cancer. It is widely believed by doctors that more men die with prostate cancer than of it. In 1999, 179,300 men were diagnosed with prostate cancer in the United States, and 37,000 died of the disease. This is roughly one death every 15 minutes across the country from prostate cancer.

Nevertheless, early detection and improving treatment options have resulted in higher survival rates—from 67 to 93 percent over the past 20 years. There was a rapid rise in the incidence of prostate cancer from 1992 to 1996 due to the introduction and wide acceptance of the prostate-specific antigen (PSA) test. During this time period, a large reservoir of men previously unscreened for prostate cancer were found to be positive for the disease. This dramatic increase in incidence has now slowed to a more normal increase in incidence driven by the aging population. Because of the widespread use of the PSA test during routine physical exams in the United States, prostate cancer is now typically diagnosed earlier in the course of the disease. Since chances of a prostate cancer cure are higher when diagnosed earlier in the course of disease, recent years have shown a steady improvement in the 5-year survival rate.

However, all the forms of primary therapy such as radical prostatectomy, external beam radiation, and brachytherapy or seed implantation have their drawbacks, and many men with early-stage prostate cancer face a difficult choice. New therapies with fewer side effects are needed to make this choice easier.

The situation is worse for men with more advanced prostate disease, for whom satisfactory treatments are still lacking. For these men, treatment options are generally not curative. Only in recent times have new targeted therapies started to enter clinical trials for prostate cancer. These new therapeutic approaches may offer some hope for men with advanced disease.

IMPROVING TREATMENT OPTIONS

An elevated PSA leads to a biopsy. If the biopsy is positive for prostate cancer and there is no evidence of lymph node or bone marrow involvement, the disease is considered to be organ-confined. There are four primary methods for dealing with organ-confined disease. They are:

- watchful waiting or no treatment
- surgery for removal of the prostate (prostatectomy)
- external beam radiation of the prostate
- brachytherapy, or the implantation of radioactive seeds directly into the prostate

Once the cancer has spread outside the prostate, additional treatment with hormone therapy or chemotherapy is an option.

SURGERY

While the cancer is confined to the prostate gland, a surgical procedure called a radical prostatectomy is often the treatment of choice. There are two kinds: radical retropubic prostatectomy, where the incision is made in the lower abdomen, and radical perineal prostatectomy, where the incision is made in the skin between the scrotum and the anus. With the first type, it is sometimes possible to avoid removing the nerves that control erections and the bladder muscles. Radical prostatectomies cure most men if the entire tumor is removed.

In 1999 about one-third of the men who were initially diagnosed with this form of cancer had surgery; there were about 65,000 prostatectomies performed. As part of the 90-minute operation, surgeons usually remove lymph nodes around the gland so that a pathologist can look for evidence of spread. Most men go home from the hospital in a few days if there are no complications. Many can work during recovery and resume unrestricted physical activity in about three weeks.

While the long-term survival rate for disease that is truly organ-confined is 95 percent five years after treatment, the complication rate is also very high. Damage to the nerve bundles near the prostate during surgery results in impotence or incontinence in as many as 60 percent of men.

Nevertheless, most men say they would have the surgery again, according to a recent large-scale study. Men who underwent radical prostatectomy for localized prostate cancer said that despite the level of urinary incontinence and sexual dysfunction, most (71.5 percent) would choose radical prostatectomy again.

Janet L. Stanford, Ph.D., from the Fred Hutchinson Cancer Research Center in Seattle, and colleagues conducted a study of over a thousand men diagnosed with primary prostate cancer. At 24 months, 59.9 percent of men reported that erections were not firm enough for sexual intercourse, and 44.2 percent were unable to have any erections. The proportion of men who reported being impotent after surgery varied according to whether a nerve-sparing procedure was attempted. The proportion of men who were able to have erections at 24 months was higher in those younger than 60 years compared with the older age groups.

This study is the most complete look at the results of prosatec-tomy in a large group of prostate cancer patients to date.

RADIATION THERAPY

Doctors have long suspected that radiation therapy helped pre-vent patients from dying of prostate cancer, but they had little sci-entific proof. Now Richard Valicenti, M.D., assistant professor of radiation oncology at Jefferson Medical College of Thomas Jefferson University in Philadelphia, and his colleagues have found the first conclusive evidence that radiation therapy helps patients with localized prostate cancer live longer. He reported his team's findings in 2000 in the *Journal of Clinical Oncology*.

Prostate cancer, the most common cancer in elderly men, tends to be a slow-growing disease. Doctors often question whether surgery or radiation provides any real benefit for the older patient.

The researchers retrospectively examined the results of 1,560 men who had received radiation therapy alone for prostate cancer. The men were among those treated between 1975 and 1995 in four separate trials conducted by the Radiation Therapy Oncology Group, a federally funded cancer clinical trials group. The average follow-up was 8 years, with some men seen for as many as 12 years.

They divided men into four categories according to the likeli-hood of having a more dangerous cancer and found that those with the worst prognoses benefited the most from receiving higher doses of radiation. After they adjusted statistically for disease sever-ity and age, they found that patients who received higher-than-usual radiation doses were 32 percent less likely to die from prostate cancer.

Dr. Valicenti, a member of Jefferson's Kimmel Cancer Center, conducted the study with his colleagues at Jefferson and other re-search centers including Wayne State University in Detroit, the University of Southern California, McAuley Health Center in Ann Arbor, Michigan, and Einstein Medical Center in Philadelphia.

External Beam Radiation

The classic radiation therapy for prostate cancer is external beam radiation, in which an X-ray machine moves around the pa-tient shooting intense X-rays or gamma rays at the prostate from different angles. Radiation therapy is generally given every week-day for eight weeks. This technique is as effective as prostatectomy in treating relatively small tumors but is not as effective in treating larger masses in the prostate. The aim of this therapy is to send a high dose of radiation to the tumor, while avoiding healthy tissue. However, even with the newer techniques, this is not always possi-ble, and, as with surgery, impotence and incontinence frequently result. In addition, the rectum is frequently damaged resulting in "leakage."

External radiation therapy can be used curatively in early can-cers, as an adjuvant therapy (with or without chemotherapy) to surgery, or to relieve symptoms if the cancer has metastasized.

Brachytherapy

In this rapidly growing procedure, a urologist and a radiation specialist place 80 to 120 radioactive pellets ("seeds") directly into the prostate where they emit radiation from within the gland. This appears to be as effective as surgery or external beam radiation. It appeals to men because of the minimal hospitalization and ab-sence of surgical scarring. There were about 25,000 brachytherapy procedures performed in this country in 1999, and this number will increase to over 100,000 as the procedure improves. Fewer men will have to undergo surgery with its high complication rate. While brachytherapy has historically been believed to produce fewer procedure-related complications, recent studies show that this may not be the case. Specifically, a study reported in the

Journal of Urology revealed that impotence might be as high as in surgery or external beam radiation.

There is not enough evidence to suggest unconditional use of brachytherapy over standard treatment of localized prostate cancer. However, researchers in Canada suggest the procedure works with their patients.

Men with low-risk prostate cancer have excellent five-year biochemical progression-free rates with standard therapies such as radical prostatectomy and external beam radiotherapy, the researchers point out. Both of these standard therapies, however, have a risk of significant long-term side effects.

Patient selection for brachytherapy is important for technical reasons as well, according to the researchers. They note that brachytherapy is currently available outside of clinical trials, but that men should be encouraged to participate in randomized trials that compare the procedure with standard treatments. Men should be as well informed as possible about the available therapies for prostate cancer and the potential adverse effects.

The study was conducted by the Genitourinary Cancer Disease Site Group of the Cancer Care Ontario Practice Guidelines Initiative.

ProstRcision

African-American men have a higher incidence of prostate cancer than do men in any other group. Their disease is usually more advanced by the time they are diagnosed. However, once they receive treatment, race is no longer a factor.

An extensive study documents that African-American men with prostate cancer who undergo a ProstRcision treatment achieve the same five-year cure rates as do white men. Published in *The Prostate Journal,* in 2000, the study was prepared by doctors at Radiotherapy Clinics of Georgia (RCOG) who developed and provide the unique ProstRcision treatment.

ProstRcision is an outpatient procedure that treats prostate cancer through a combination of seed implants followed by conformal beam radiation. Conformal beam radiation is a three-dimensional technique that provides greater accuracy than other techniques. ProstRcision has produced the highest cure rate ever published after radiation for prostate cancer—88 percent after five and seven years—and with the least amount of complications. Most men retain complete sexual function, and none have urinary incontinence.

The study was conducted by Drs. W. Hamilton Williams, Frank Critz, James B. Benton, Keith Levinson, Walter Falconer, Emerson Harrison, Clinton T. Holladay, and David A. Holladay. Over 2.5 million data points on all men who have received the ProstRcision treatment over the last 20 years make up RCOG's database, the foundation of the ProstRcision treatment program. This database, one of the largest in the country, is used for clinical research as well as to help train other doctors and to determine how patients are to be treated for prostate cancer.

Intensity Modulated Radiation Therapy

A technique called intensity modulated radiation therapy, or IMRT, subjects the prostate to more conformal radiation than standard radiation treatment. IMRT is often used in combination with brachytherapy.

Dr. Glen Gejerman, clinical director of the Department of Radiation Oncology at Hackensack University Medical Center in New Jersey, heads a team of specialists that has been studying the effects of IMRT. They found that men undergoing therapy for organ-confined prostate cancer no longer have to suffer from side effects such as rectal bleeding and diarrhea.

There are a number of things that the IMRT and the Theraseed palladium seed implant have achieved, according to Dr. Gejerman. The dose directly to the prostate can be escalated, and this has been shown to increase the chances of cure.

The study is an analysis of 65 prostate cancer patients treated with IMRT and seed implantation. The results were presented at the annual meeting of the American Radium Society in London.

According to Dr. Gejerman, IMRT is no longer just theoretical but is in clinical use. Curative doses of radiation are being delivered to the prostate without the typical side effects, he reported.

Since palladium radioactive seeds are placed directly into the prostate gland, the surrounding rectum and bladder receive very little radiation. What the study means is that prostate cancer patients can get a higher dose to the prostate and a lower dose to the bladder and rectum with fewer side effects, according to Dr. Gejerman.

The overwhelming worry for patients when they consider surgery for prostate cancer is whether they can be cured. Once they are assured of that, the next question is how it is going to affect their lifestyles. Men are greatly concerned that they may have to constantly run to the bathroom to urinate, or have diarrhea. They don't want to be embarrassed. With IMRT and palladium seed implantation therapy there is a good chance of avoiding such problems, according to Dr. Gejerman.

While the study was limited to the initial 65 patients treated, a total of 200 patients have been treated without showing any rectal side effects. Dr. Stephen Strum, an oncologist/hematologist in Marina Del Ray, California, said he believed IMRT would soon become the standard radiation therapy approach, not only for prostate cancer, but also for all tumor types.

Many cancer centers are treating prostate cancer with the combination of external beam therapy and a palladium seed implant, but Hackensack is said to be the only facility in the country doing IMRT and seed implantation in large numbers. There are a limited number of physicians experienced at treating prostate cancer with IMRT. Over 200 patients have been treated with IMRT at the Prostate Cancer Institute of Hackensack University Medical Center. The institute has treated more patients with IMRT in combination with brachytherapy than any other program in the country.

Daily treatments are Monday through Friday over an eight-week period. Treatments take 20 minutes to deliver and have no immediate aftereffects. During radiation seed implant treatment, doctors implant tiny palladium radioactive seeds, each about the size of a grain of rice, directly into the prostate gland using ultrasound guidance. Once inside, the seeds target and destroy cancerous cells, while minimizing exposure to surrounding tissues.

Getting Radiation Therapy

Radiation oncologists and urologists don't always agree on treatments, according to a survey of the specialists who treat most of the approximately 180,000 new cases of prostate cancer diagnosed each year. The study, sponsored by the U.S. Agency for Healthcare Research and Quality (AHRQ), reports that the two groups of specialists largely agree that radical prostate surgery, external beam radiotherapy, and brachytherapy are potentially lifesaving treatments for localized prostate cancer in men whose normal life expectancy is ten years or longer. But not surprisingly, urologists prefer surgery and radiation oncologists prefer radiation therapy.

More than nine of every ten urologists questioned said they considered prostate surgery better than radiation therapy for men with a life expectancy of ten years or more, while 72 percent of the radiation oncologists indicated that they believed radiotherapy worked as well as radical prostatectomy for such men.

To date, randomized clinical trials have not proven that aggressive treatment of prostate cancer with either surgery or radiotherapy improves patient outcomes, but neither have they proven that the two therapies are ineffective.

Many newly diagnosed prostate cancer patients have a difficult time choosing the best treatment. According to AHRQ director John M. Eisenberg, M.D., a doctor's clinical judgment is based on scientific evidence. But the research findings on outcomes are not always decisive enough to support the evidence.

The best way to help the patient is to schedule consultations with a member of each specialty before making a decision. This may be the best way to get a balanced view of treatment options, according to Michael J. Barry, M.D., of the Medical Practices Evaluation Center at Massachusetts General Hospital.

The researchers also found that:

- Both groups of physicians generally agreed on the probability of complications from all three therapies and agreed that prostatectomy is more likely than radiotherapy to cause incontinence and sexual dysfunction.
- Fewer than 25 percent in either group said they would recommend watchful waiting to men with unaggressive tumors despite that fact that such patients appear to have a normal life expectancy without aggressive treatment.
- About 40 percent would recommend androgen deprivation to men with the most aggressive tumors and highest PSA levels.
- Despite insufficient data on the long-term effects of brachytherapy, members of both specialties generally thought it at least as good as external beam radiation. Urologists seemed to be slightly more positive about brachytherapy than external beam radiotherapy.

The survey analysis was conducted by researchers from the University of Massachusetts, Massachusetts General Hospital, and the University of Connecticut Health Center. Details are in "Comparison of Treatment Recommendations by Urologists and Radiation Oncologists for Men with Clinically Localized Prostate Cancer," in the June 28, 2000, issue of the *Journal of the American Medical Association*.

HORMONE THERAPY

Because the growth of prostate cancer is usually dependent on male hormones, manipulation of the hormone levels in the body can relieve symptoms and reverse tumor growth. The exact cause of prostate cancer is unknown, but it is thought to be related to the stimulatory action of the male sex hormone testosterone, and as men age, they are more vulnerable to the long-term effects of testosterone. It's similar to the risk for women of estrogen and breast cancer.

Drugs called luteinizing hormone–releasing hormone (LHRH)

agonists, such as Leupron and Zoladex, that decrease the amount of male hormones are the main hormone suppressors used in prostate cancer today. Antiandrogens, such as flutamide (Eulexin), bicalutamide (Casodex), and nilutamide (Nilandron), are sometimes used to block the body's ability to use any remaining androgens.

Other hormonal drugs, including megestrol acetate (Megace) and medroxyprogesterone (Depo-Provera), and ketoconazole (Nizoral), which acts as an antiandrogen, are used if first-line hormonal therapies lose their effectiveness. Remissions with hormone therapy are generally temporary, lasting two to three years.

Casodex

A recent example of the use of hormonal regulation to control prostate cancer is Casodex. Casodex is an oral hormonal medication that interferes with the ability of prostate cancer cells to use male hormones to grow. Casodex is a nonsteroidal antiandrogen that works by blocking the action of androgens, such as testosterone, at the cellular level.

In data presented from the largest prostate cancer clinical trial program in the world, Casodex 150 mg tablets was shown to significantly reduce (42 percent) the risk of disease progression in men with localized prostate cancer.

The program was undertaken to study the effect of Casodex 150 mg as an immediate treatment for early prostate cancer and was designed on the same premise as the adjuvant trials of tamoxifen in breast cancer. The results from the Early Prostate Cancer Trial (EPC) program were presented at the American Society of Clinical Oncology annual meeting in San Francisco in 2001.

The EPC is an international program composed of three clinical trials. The program, which began in 1995, is the largest prostate cancer trial program ever conducted and includes over 8,000 patients from 23 countries around the world, including North America, Europe including Scandinavia, South Africa, Australia, and Mexico. The program is designed to determine whether adding Casodex 150 mg to standard care (radical prostatectomy, radiation therapy, or watchful waiting) can reduce the risk of disease progression when compared to standard therapy alone, in patients whose cancer has not spread to other organs.

According to Manfred Wirth, M.D., chairman of the Department of Urology at the Technical University of Dresden in Germany, and one of the lead investigators for the EPC program, results so far indicate that men with earlier-stage prostate cancer may reduce the risk of their disease progressing if they take Casodex 150 mg as immediate or adjuvant therapy. William A. See, M.D., professor and chief, Division of Urology, Medical College of Wisconsin, Milwaukee, and a lead investigator for the EPC program in the United States, called the results encouraging.

Casodex 150 mg is not approved for use in the United States. However, the lower-dose 50 mg tablet is available for combination therapy with a luteinizing hormone–releasing hormone analogue (LHRH-A), such as Zoladex, for the treatment of Stage D2 metastatic prostate cancer.

Hormones and Radiation

In1998 the FDA approved Zoladex (goserelin acetate implant) in combination with the antiandrogen flutamide prior to and during radiation therapy for the management of early stages of prostate cancer. This makes Zoladex the first and only hormonal treatment in its class approved for combination treatment against early cancer confined to the prostate gland.

The effects of Zoladex in combination with flutamide plus radiation therapy were studied in 466 patients compared to radiation alone in men with locally confined prostate cancer. Conducted by the Radiation Therapy Oncology Group, the multicenter study showed that disease-free survival was significantly increased in the group with combined surgery. Combination therapy also reduced distant spread of the disease (27 percent versus 36 percent at four years).

This type of hormone therapy causes testosterone production to stop. The therapy is administered through an injection into the fat just below the skin of the abdomen, where the biodegradable implant slowly dissolves, delivering the drug continuously over a four-hour period.

CHEMOTHERAPY

Taxotere and Estramustine Phosphate

Combination chemotherapy with Taxotere and estramustine phosphate is a highly active treatment for men with advanced prostate cancer. This new regimen could become important for men whose disease continues to advance despite treatment.

Daniel P. Petrylak, M.D., assistant professor of medicine, Columbia University College of Physicians and Surgeons, presented these findings at the 36th annual meeting of the American Society of Clinical Oncology in 2001. Dr. Petrylak is also director of the Genitourinary Oncology Program, Columbia Presbyterian Medical Center, in New York.

The average age of the 37 men in this trial was 69 and they were very sick, with 33 of the men experiencing bone metastases. Estramustine 280 mg was given orally three times a day for five days. Taxotere was given on the second day of the treatment course by one-hour infusion. Patients had failed primary hormonal and secondary hormonal therapy, which included cortisone, ketoconazole, and flutamide.

After one year in the trial, 77 percent of the men were alive and 25 had their PSA levels drop by more than 50 percent. In 14 men, the PSA decreased by 80 percent or more. The median duration of response was 18 weeks.

Dr. Petrylak said the trial was prompted by laboratory data demonstrating synergy between estramustine and Taxotere.

Exisulind

Columbia Presbyterian researchers have found that a new drug may be an option for slowing tumor growth in men with advanced prostate cancer. The study is the first of its kind to show a significant effect of a new class of drugs that may stabilize progressive, recurrent disease in men with advanced prostate cancer.

The principal investigator was Dr. Erik Goluboff, assistant professor of urology at Columbia University College of Physicians and Surgeons and director of urology at the Allen Pavilion of the New York–Presbyterian Hospital. The evidence indicates that the drug exisulind, developed by Cell Pathways, the company that funded the trial, increases the rate of programmed cell death in cancer cells without damaging normal cells. The cancerous cells die and can no longer keep dividing and multiplying, which stops the cancer from growing. These drugs do not produce most of the adverse reactions or serious side effects normally associated with chemotherapy.

For 12 months, the researchers followed 96 prostate cancer patients who had had their prostates removed. All had rising prostate-specific antigen (PSA) levels indicating recurrent disease. Half received exisulind and half were given a placebo.

The exisulind reduced the growth of prostate cancer in men with progressive, recurrent disease, thereby possibly providing long-term disease control with low incidence of side effects otherwise unattainable for this patient group, according to Dr. Goluboff.

ABT-627 and Clodronate

In about 30 percent of men with prostate cancer, the disease eventually metastasizes in the bone. A first study included 244 men in this condition who did not yet have pain and other symptoms. They received an oral drug, ABT-627 (atrasentan), or a placebo. Those treated with the drug had longer intervals from the time of metastasis until the pain developed. The drug also doubled the time it took for their PSA level to rise.

According to Michael Carducci, M.D., the lead study author and assistant professor of oncology at Johns Hopkins University, this is exciting because it suggests that a pill with few toxic side effects can delay the time until additional systemic treatment is needed.

Another study, conducted by British researchers, found that of

311 men with advanced prostate cancer that spread to the bone, those who used oral clodronate also had a delay in the pain.

A Phase III trial result suggests they survive seven months longer.

Taxotere

Weekly treatment with Taxotere (docetaxel) significantly reduces bone pain resulting from progressive prostate cancer while also decreasing PSA levels. These results enhance the quality of life for patients, according to researchers at Oregon Health Sciences University (OHSU).

Tomasz Beer, M.D., an oncologist at the OHSU School of Medicine and lead investigator of the study, said, "Our results suggest that weekly docetaxel not only represents an effective and well-tolerated agent for relieving bone pain in these patients but also reduces disease activity by means of a decrease in PSA levels."

The 25 men who participated in the trial had an advanced form of cancer known as hormone-refractory prostate cancer and also experienced bone pain. These patients all had progressive disease despite standard hormonal therapy including androgen withdrawal. The men received weekly infusions of docetaxel for six weeks, followed by a two-week rest period. The eight-week regimen was continued until there was evidence of disease progression.

Forty-four percent of patients achieved significant relief of pain without an increase in use of pain medication. OHSU is an academic medical center in Portland, Oregon, featuring schools of medicine, nursing, and dentistry. An outstanding research facility, OHSU is among the top 30 institutions funded by the National Institutes of Health.

Targeted Bone Chemotherapy

Survival can be increased among men who respond to chemotherapy for advanced prostate cancer if specific therapy is targeted at sites of bone metastases. In a Phase II trial, Dr. Shi-Ming

Tu and colleagues at the Department of Genitourinary Medical Oncology, University of Texas M. D. Anderson Cancer Center in Houston, reported on the value of bone-targeted consolidation therapy in patients with advanced androgen-independent cancer of the prostate.

They studied 103 patients who received induction chemotherapy, consisting of ketoconazole and doxorubicin alternating with estramustine and vinblastine. After two or three cycles of induction chemotherapy, the clinicians randomly assigned 72 patients who were clinically responding, or stable, to receive doxorubicin every week for six weeks with or without one dosage of strontium-89 (Sr-89). Sixty-two of the 103 patients (60 percent) had a 50 percent or greater reduction in serum PSA, and 43 patients (42 percent) had an 80 percent or greater reduction. In addition, 49 patients (52 percent) had no more bone pain.

The average survival for all 103 patients was 17.5 months. For the 36 patients randomly assigned to receive Sr-89 and doxorubicin, the median survival time was 27.7 months, compared to 16.8 for the 36 who received doxorubicin alone.

Researchers say these results support the hypothesis that bone-targeted therapy can alter the natural history of patients with advanced androgen-independent cancer of the prostate. The consolidation and induction chemotherapy regimens were both developed at M. D. Anderson Cancer Center.

EXPERIMENTAL TREATMENTS

While molecular research and biotech drugs have advanced to the stage of clinical use for some cancers, they are still only in the experimental stage for prostate cancer.

Targeted Virus

In September 2000 cancer researchers began testing an experimental drug in men with metastatic prostate cancer who failed hormone therapy. The drug, CV787, kills targeted cancer cells, leaving normal, or noncancerous, cells unharmed. Scientists at Calydon, a Silicon Valley biotechnology company, engineered CV787 as an oncolytic (cancer-killing) virus that kills human prostate cancer cells 10,000 times more frequently than normal cells. This targeting is significantly better than chemotherapy, which kills only two to six cancer cells for each normal cell incidentally killed. It is also better than radiation therapy, which kills all rapidly dividing cells indiscriminately.

It has been reported that Calydon's CV787, alone or in combination with chemotherapy, might offer novel treatment options for both hormone-sensitive and hormone-insensitive metastatic prostate cancer.

Calydon has discovered a gene, prostate-specific enhancer (PSE), which controls PSA production in the body. PSE has been genetically engineered into an adenovirus (a type of cold virus) that infects only PSA-producing cells.

Intravenous CV787 is being tested at three medical centers: the University of California at San Francisco, Johns Hopkins Oncology Center in Baltimore, and the University of Wisconsin at Madison. The Phase I and II trials enrolled about 48 men to find out whether CV787 given intravenously is safe and how it affects the PSA level. An earlier trial at Johns Hopkins in 20 men with recurrent disease confined to the prostate showed encouraging results, according to David B. Karpf, M.D., vice president of Clinical and Regulatory Affairs at Calydon.

Calydon is engaged in the discovery, development, and commercialization of novel virus-based therapeutics for cancer. The company is able to create tumor-specific viruses that replicate in and kill targeted cancer cells, leaving noncancer cells unharmed. Calydon is in Phase I and II development for its prostate cancer therapeutics at many sites in the United States. For more information on Calydon's clinical program, visit their web site at www.calydon.com/cgi/overview.php or www.calydon.com.

Targeted Virus and Radiation

Calydon is also testing a virus for use with radiation therapy. This drug, CN706, was tested on 20 men who failed conventional radiation therapy. Phase I and II study results in October 2000 indicated antitumor activity, and the men were able to tolerate the drug well.

CN706 is administered by a modified prostate brachytherapy technique and was tested at five different dose levels without adverse affects. Four of the 11 men given the highest doses showed a 50 percent or greater drop in their PSA levels for at least four weeks. Three men had a partial response that lasted for at least nine months. These studies are continuing.

Patient-specific vaccines

A team of Johns Hopkins Oncology Center researchers had developed a vaccine that helps strengthen the body's immune system against prostate cancer, according to a study published in the journal *Cancer Research*. The study showed a vaccine can trigger the immune system to fight cancer the way it fights infection. Researchers injected a genetically engineered vaccine into 11 prostate cancer patients, whose disease was still spreading after their prostates were removed. In 8 of the 11 men, tumors shrank, according to the study. The experiment produced not only the release of T cells as researchers had hoped, but also the production of antibodies against cancer. Both are key weapons of the immune system.

In the Hopkins study, scientists removed tumors from each of the 11 patients, chopped up the tissue, and grew them on laboratory culture dishes. A gene called GMF-CSF, which produces a protein that alerts tissues to the presence of foreign substances, was inserted into the cancer cells. The vaccine was then irradiated to prevent any further cancerous growth and injected into the patients' thighs, like a flu shot. The study was funded by the National Cancer Institute, the Department of Defense Prostate Cancer Initiative.

Non-patient-specific vaccine

Because preliminary studies were encouraging, clinical trials for GVAX for prostate expanded in 2001. The second generation

GVAX is being tested by the Cell Genesys Corporation in a Phase I/II clinical trial in prostate cancer patients. Unlike specific vaccine made from a patient's own cells, this is allogeneic (not patient-specific) and involves genetic modification of cell lines which have been irradiated and modified.

This approach makes it possible to manufacture a vaccine that can be used "off the shelf" to treat any patient and could be commercialized much like a traditional pharmaceutical product. This trial is being conducted at Johns Hopkins Medical Institutions and results were reported in 1998.

Disease stabilization and a decrease in the rate of rise of PSA levels were observed in 11 of 15 patients. Two patients experienced a greater than 50 percent decrease in PSA levels, in one case continuing after six months.

Stephen A. Sherwin, M.D., chairman and CEO of Cell Genesys, said the company was encouraged by initial findings and would advance the clinical development program as rapidly as possible. He said the cancer vaccines have shown objective evidence of antitumor activity in all five types of cancer in which they have been tested.

In the Phase II study, a six-month treatment with GVAX, men with prostate cancer received an initial priming dose followed by 12 biweekly booster doses using either a low dose or a threefold higher dose regimen. No other cancer therapies were given. The doses were administered by intradermal injection into the skin of the arms and legs, with few side effects.

Cell Genesys's most advanced therapeutic program is the GVAX cancer vaccines, which are treatment vaccines that have been safely administered to well over 300 patients to date. Cell Genesys's non-patient-specific cancer vaccines are made of irradiated tumor cells which have been genetically modified to secrete granulocyte-macrophage colony stimulating factor (GMF-CSF), a hormone which plays a key role in stimulating the body's immune response to vaccines.

The vaccines are then administered under the skin, potentially stimulating a systemic immune response that targets and destroys tumor cells that persist or recur following surgery and/or radiation therapy. Cell Genesys believes that an important advantage of GVAX cancer vaccines is that they are "whole-cell," vaccines which don't require that specific antigens (proteins on the surface of cells) be identified prior to developing the vaccines.

GVAX has now been reported to show evidence of antitumor activity in humans in all five types of cancer tested to date—including prostate cancer, pancreatic cancer, lung cancer, melanoma, and kidney cancer—suggesting that GVAX may be applicable to multiple types of cancer.

Antigen Vaccines

Dendreon Corporation's Provenge, a therapeutic vaccine for the treatment of prostate cancer, is currently being tested in two Phase III clinical trials. Dendreon is focusing on the discovery and development of immunologically based therapy for cancer.

"Through the use of antigen discovery, antigen engineering and dendritic cell technologies, Dendreon develops therapeutic vaccines designed to induce cell-mediated immunity—the body's key defense against cancer," said Christopher S. Henney, Ph.D., chief executive officer and chairman of the Board of Directors.

"The antigen component of Provenge is derived from the gene encoding a marker for prostate cancer, prostatic acid phosphatase, which is found in approximately 95 percent of prostate cancers," Dr. Henney said.

Progenics Pharmaceuticals and Cytogen Corporation also have a new vaccine for prostate cancer. It is directed against the prostate-specific membrane antigen (PSMA), the unique protein found on the surface of prostate cancer cells. The vaccine is designed to stimulate the patient's immune system to recognize and destroy the cancer cells. The companies reported preclinical findings in September 2000.

"Based on our recent scientific advances, we have successfully produced a vaccine candidate that faithfully mimics the PSMA structure expressed on prostate cancer cells," said William C. Olson, Ph.D., senior director of research and development at Progenics.

The companies are also developing monoclonal antibodies and virus vaccines to bring to clinical trials.

Other Emerging Treatments

Chemotherapy combined with androgen deprivation is being studied as front-line therapy in advanced cancer. Longer survival has been seen in many trials.

A new form of gene therapy for men with prostate cancers that are hard to treat is being studied at three medical centers. The Cleveland Clinic said this trial will involve injecting genetic material into prostate glands of men with cancers that are hard to cure with surgery or radiation. Dr. Eric Klein, head of urologic oncology and coordinator of the study at the Cleveland Clinic, said the treatment may be the wave of the future. The material is leuvectin and is made up of DNA. It produces the protein interleukin-2 (IL-2).

WHERE TO FIND INFORMATION ABOUT PROSTATE CANCER

The Association for the Cure of Cancer of the Prostate (CaPCURE)
Web site: www.capcure.org

Founded in 1993 by Michael Milken, this organization has become the largest source of private money raised for research into prostate cancer. The web is a good source of current clinical trials. The trials are listed by location and by type of treatment.

Man to Man
American Cancer Society
1599 Clifton Road, NE
Atlanta, GA 30329
Telephone: 800-ACS-2345
Web site: www.cancer.org/m2m/m2m/html

This group has chapters all over the country to help men deal with the emotional fallout of having prostate cancer. It offers community-based education, discussion, and support, and is for men recently diagnosed as well as long-term survivors. Man to Man helps men learn how to communicate with their doctors and keeps them informed about latest treatments. In addition to educational programs, it offers social activities.

ONGOING CLINICAL TRIALS FOR PROSTATE CANCER

There are literally hundreds of clinical trials in various stages of development around the world. To list them all here would be misleading because by the time you read this book, some trials may have closed and many others may have opened. Clinical trials have specific eligibility requirements that may eliminate many cancer patients. The few trials listed here are only a sampling of the trials that may be open to you. The best way to locate clinical trials appropriate for your situation is to ask your doctor, check the web sites listed in Chapter 4, and call the biotech companies listed in Appendix C.

1. A Phase I study of the HSV-tk gene in men with recurrence of prostate cancer after radiation therapy is being conducted at Baylor College of Medicine and the Methodist Hospital. The principal investigator is Dr. Brian J. Miles. Baylor has a number of protocols that might be of interest to men with prostate cancer. For information call 713-798-4079 or e-mail Linda Higgins at lhiggins@bcm.tmc.edu.
2. An angiogenesis inhibitor, AG3340, made by Agouron Pharmaceuticals is in Phase II and III clinical trials for men with advanced prostate cancer. In rodents, this drug potently inhibits angiogenesis (the formation of new blood vessels that feed growing tumors), tumor growth, and metastasis. It also enhances the antitumor activity of certain conventional chemotherapy agents. Phase I studies have shown AG3340 to be well tolerated at the doses to be administered in the trials,

which have an initial Phase II dose evaluation period. In a randomized trial, patients with advanced hormone-refractory prostate cancer will receive AG3340 in tablet form in combination with Novantrone (mitoxantrone) and prednisone. The primary objective of this study is to evaluate time to symptomatic progression of disease.

3. Cell Genesys is conducting trials with about 30 patients for its vaccine GVAX. Following a prostatectomy, patients whose PSA is still rising will receive multiple vaccinations of GVAX. Expanded clinical trials of GVAX in prostate cancer were expected to begin in 2001. For information call 650-425-4542 or www.cellgenesys.com.

4. Calydon is sponsoring a dose-finding trial of CV787, adenovirus, in men with locally recurrent cancer following radiotherapy.

CHAPTER 9

▼

BREAKTHROUGH TREATMENTS FOR LUNG CANCER

Lung cancer is the leading cause of cancer-related death in both men and women in the United States, with approximately 160,000 deaths each year. It accounts for 28 percent of all cancer deaths, according to the National Cancer Institute (NCI). Most cases occur between the ages of 60 and 80. During 2000, approximately 177,000 new primary lung cancers were diagnosed in the United States. About 25 percent will undergo surgery.

Here are some interesting ways to think about it:

- If lung cancer death rates were equivalent to prostate or breast cancer at about 20 percent, then 110,000 people a year would not die.
- The way to get the death rate down is to find a diagnostic test to detect lung cancer earlier.

Despite continued advances in diagnostic techniques, advances in chemotherapy and radiation protocols, and new understanding of fundamental molecular biology, the survival rate for lung cancer has shown only minimal improvement over the past several decades.

By the time of diagnosis, the cancer will already have metastasized in two-thirds of the patients. Conventional treatment for lung cancer has been to remove all or part of the lung. In later stages this is followed with chemotherapy and sometimes radiation. The two-year survival rate for people with Stage III disease is 20 percent and goes to less than 5 percent once it reaches Stage IV.

However, with new molecular approaches to the disease, it has become possible to understand the genetic and biological properties of cancer cells. This may lead to better therapies for survival in the near future. The lung cancer fight is going on at the molecular level. Drugs that attack the EGFR (epidermal growth factor receptors) can also have therapeutic activity in lung cancer. Patients will be able to experience a regression of tumors never before seen with standard chemotoxic agents and radiation. AstraZeneca has been developing a drug called Iressa. OSI Pharmaceuticals has a new targeted therapy called Tarceva (OSI774), which also acts by blocking EGFR.

The promising new chemotherapy drugs are paclitaxel (Taxol), topotecan, and vinorelbine. In the first study of its kind, a team of British researchers found that three courses of a frequently used chemotherapy regimen—mitomycin C, vinblastine, and cisplatin—achieved the same clinical benefit as six courses in patients with advanced non–small cell lung cancer (NSCLC), the most common kind. This study was reported in the *Journal of Clinical Oncology* in March 2001. For many patients, the side effects of the sustained longer use of chemotherapy are extremely unpleasant. The study showed that there was no substantial difference in survival times of patients who had three or six months of chemotherapy, but the side effects such as fatigue were significantly decreased with the shorter course.

Today there are many clinical trials in progress that treat the disease with new biotech therapies, most in combination with conventional chemotherapy. Radiation therapy has also improved with a new technique called respiratory gating that can pinpoint the radiation beam more precisely without the contamination of surrounding lung tissue that normally occurs because the lungs move with every breath.

ANGIOGENESIS INHIBITORS

Years ago, when desperate cancer patients went to other countries to buy shark cartilage, they were pitied as being easily duped because of their condition. Even some alternative healers, not usually so averse to "natural" remedies, considered shark cartilage a pipe dream. Today, shark cartilage is the source for Neovastat, an angiogenesis inhibitor, and is marketed all over the world. Another "natural" part of the dog shark, the tissue from the liver, is the basis of squalamine, a similar drug currently in clinical trials throughout the world.

Roy Levitt, M.D., president and CEO of Geneara (formerly Magainin Pharmaceuticals), said, "We have been impressed that many outstanding investigators have demonstrated the potent antiangiogenic effects of squalamine, in many different model systems. We also remain encouraged by the early clinical results with squalamine, in both our lung and ovarian cancer trials." Squalamine is being developed to treat a variety of cancers.

Neovastat is the lead antiangiogenesis agent made by Aeterna, a Quebec company. It is currently in clinical trials for lung, kidney, and ovarian cancer and multiple myeloma. Angiogenesis is implicated in the development of more than twenty diseases, including cancer, psoriasis, and age-related macular degeneration.

Cartilage has been studied for its potential to inhibit the development of new blood vessels, which tumors require to grow, as well as acting directly to slow tumor cell growth. The precise factors responsible for these effects are not yet known, but since cartilage accounts for approximately 6 percent of the body weight in sharks, they are an excellent source of these antiangiogenic factors. An extraction and purification method was developed by Aeterna. One of these fractions, Neovastat (formerly AE941), has been used in the laboratory in petri dishes as well as in live tumor-bearing animals. The results indicate an antitumor potential without any signs of toxicity.

Early in 1997, a Phase I study of Neovastat was implemented for patients with solid tumors of the lung, breast, and prostate. The present study extends this potentially effective treatment to patients with any type of solid tumor who have no other therapies available. (See the list of clinical trials on page 136.)

Some patients have been taking Neovastat continuously for almost four years. The only thing they complain about is the fishy smell. A young patient who failed chemotherapy and had metastatic lung cancer with multiple lung nodules responded well and extended her life for two years rather than the few months expected with lung cancer.

Aeterna Laboratories has been selected by the National Cancer Institute, a branch of the National Institutes of Health (NIH), to test Neovastat in pivotal Phase III trials to evaluate its effectiveness in the treatment of cancer. Neovastat was to be given to several hundred cancer patients around the country. Such studies are of great importance for medical oncologists to evaluate the value of an antiangiogenic agent like Neovastat in the treatment of cancer in combination with conventional therapies, according to Dr. William Evans, medical director and CEO of the Ottawa Regional Cancer Centre and member of Aeterna's Scientific Advisory Board.

Dr. Eric Dupont, president and CEO of Aeterna, cited NCI's involvement in the clinical development program of Neovastat as important for his company because it moves the project closer to the submission of a new drug application.

Neovastat is a liquid cartilage extract that has been tested on over 450 patients with advanced cancer in the United States and Canada. Phase I and Phase II clinical trials in lung and prostate cancer have established the drug's excellent safety and tolerability at all dosage levels tested. In fact, no drug-related serious adverse events have been reported to date, which allows the studies to proceed at the highest dose.

ANTISENSE THERAPY AND CHEMOTHERAPY

Gemzar

The FDA approved Gemzar, an antisense drug made by Eli Lilly and Co., for use in combination with cisplatin, a commonly used anticancer drug, for the first-line treatment of inoperable, locally advanced, or metastatic NSCLC, the most common type. This drug has already been approved as a single agent for the first-line treatment of locally advanced or metastatic pancreatic cancer. Currently, Gemzar is approved in more than 65 countries for lung, pancreatic, or other types of cancer. It is available in more than 55 countries for lung cancer.

Gemzar was featured in 221 scientific papers at the American Society of Clinical Oncology (ASCO) in 2001.

"It was just prior to ASCO five years ago that we officially received FDA approval to market Gemzar in the United States for the treatment of locally advanced or metastatic pancreatic cancer," said Garry Nicholson, executive director of Lilly Oncology in the United States. "Today Gemzar is also approved in the United States for treatment of non–small cell lung cancer, and it is approved in more than 70 countries for treating these devastating types of cancer. It is one of the most highly sought-after combination agents in clinical research across a variety of tumor types."

Researchers from this country and abroad presented data from Phase II and III studies in which Gemzar was combined with or compared with other treatment regimens.

"Most lung cancer therapies will include either carboplatin or cisplatin, but researchers are also looking at non-platinum combinations using agents such as Gemzar, Taxol, and Taxotere," said Jorge Otero, M.D., of Lilly's Gemzar product team.

"When left untreated, advanced lung cancer can take the lives of patients within four months," said Alan Sandler, M.D., assistant professor of medicine at Indiana University School of Medicine and lead investigator for a Gemzar trial. "Our study showed that 39 percent of patients who received Gemzar plus cisplatin were still alive after one year compared with only 28 percent of patients who received cisplatin alone. These results are both statistically and clinically significant."

The FDA's decision to approve Gemzar for non–small cell lung cancer was based in part on results from a large Phase III trial that showed a significant survival advantage among those who received the combination regimen of Gemzar and cisplatin compared with patients who received cisplatin alone. The study evaluated 522 patients with advanced NSCLC at 39 sites in North America and Europe.

"Without question, this study confirms that the combination regimen of Gemzar-cisplatin is significantly better than cisplatin alone when measuring survival time, disease progression and objective tumor response," Sandler said.

Isis 3521

Isis 3521, an antisense anticancer drug, continues to demonstrate prolonged survival and time to progression of disease in people with NSCLC, according to Phase I and II studies. Clinical trial results on Isis 3521, in combination with standard chemotherapy in patients with Stages IIIB and IV NSCLC, were presented at the ASCO meeting in 2001. Alan Yuen, M.D., assistant professor of medicine at Stanford University, summarized the findings.

To date, the median survival time of people in the trial is 15.9 months. Typical median survival of patients receiving standard chemotherapy alone is approximately 8 months. The median time to progression of disease for patients involved in the study is 6.3 months. Of the 48 patients who were evaluated for response, 81 percent improved through tumor responses or stable disease.

"These data continue to look very promising for patients with non–small cell lung cancer," said Dr. Yuen. "Because PKC-alpha, the target for Isis 3521, is important in several critical tumor cell processes, the drug may be enhancing the effects of chemotherapy in a number of ways. These results are particularly meaningful in a patient population that is in great need of new therapies and improved quality of life."

Based on results observed earlier in this trial, Isis initiated a randomized Phase III trial of the drug in October 2000. The 600-patient Phase III trial is currently enrolling and will evaluate the ability of Isis 3521 to safely prolong life when combined with carboplatin and paclitaxel. "We continue to be excited by the strength of these data at this stage of maturity, and are hopeful that additional studies of Isis 3521 will demonstrate the drug's ability to help people with lung cancer," said Andrew Dorr, M.D., Isis vice president and chief medical officer. "Our Phase III trial, if successful, will be a significant advance in that direction. We believe that Isis 3521, an antisense drug, may represent a new approach to target-specific therapy in the treatment of cancer."

PATIENT-SPECIFIC VACCINES

Cell Genesys announced early positive results from its ongoing Phase I and II GVAX lung cancer vaccine clinical trial. A man who had failed standard chemotherapy had a complete response to vaccine treatment with the disappearance of all previously detected lung cancer tumors. He was treated by John Nemunaitis, M.D., at U.S. Oncology in Dallas, Texas, one of eight clinical trial sites. Based on this success, Cell Genesys has enrolled up to 80 patients in its Phase I/II trials. Results were expected by mid-2001.

GVAX trials are evaluating both early-stage lung cancer patients and those at high risk for recurrence, and advanced-stage patients who have failed other therapies. An earlier Phase I/II trial of GVAX lung cancer vaccine in patients with advanced non–small cell lung cancer showed antitumor immunity in 18 of 25 patients. These two trials have employed a patient-specific vaccine prepared from the patient's own tumor cells. This is done in an overnight process that can be carried out at the hospital where the patient is treated.

Cell Genesys plans to develop a *non*-patient-specific GVAX vaccine, too. Others have reported encouraging results in initial clinical trials in prostate and pancreatic cancer.

RADIATION THERAPY

Repiratory Gating

Do you remember the TV image of the truck crossing the bridge in Iraq during the Gulf War? Remember how those crosshairs from the airborne gunner overhead zeroed in on that truck and followed it across the bridge? Then how the bomb followed those crosshairs right into the truck and exploded and was completely destroyed? Well, that's what a new technique to fight cancer does using a radiation beam that homes right in on the tumor. That technique is called respiratory gating. It could save your life.

In late September 2000, St. Vincent's Comprehensive Cancer Center in New York treated its first patient using the respiratory gating technique. Five radiation beams were pointed at the lung tumor while the patient was breathing normally. Dr. Anthony Berson, chairman of radiation oncology, said, "This technique represents the latest advancement in nonsurgical cancer treatment." It is made possible by a combination of medical imaging, 3D simulation, treatment beam shaping, and respiratory monitoring.

This quantum leap in computer-aided cancer treatment provides precise and powerful treatment of lung and other cancers—with virtually no damage to healthy tissue. With respiratory gating you can breathe naturally and remain comfortable during treatment. And it has virtually no side effects.

Radiation therapy uses penetrating beams of high-energy waves called X-rays or gamma rays. Radiation injures or destroys cells in the tumor by damaging their genetic material, making it impossible for these cells to continue to grow. Because cancer cells grow and divide more rapidly than most of the normal cells around them, radiation therapy can successfully treat many kinds of cancer. Small amounts of surrounding normal cells may also be affected by radiation, but unlike cancer cells, most of them recover from the effects of radiation and are able to function properly.

Respiratory gating is the process of turning on the radiation beam as a function of a patient's breathing cycle. When you breathe, your internal organs move as much as several centimeters, causing the tumors to move in and out of the radiation treatment field. Using respiratory gating, your radiation treatment is synchronized to your individual breathing pattern, limiting the radiation beam to coming on only during one specific part of the breathing cycle and targeting the tumor only when it is in the optimum range. This technique reduces potential complications and side effects, allowing for higher doses and better outcomes.

Why deliver high doses of radiation? Some aggressive cancers—like lung cancer tumors—may require higher radiation doses for better control. Higher radiation doses can be delivered only if the dose to normal tissues can be kept to safe levels. Stereotactic radiosurgery in combination with respiratory gating makes this possible.

Computer-guided imaging, simulation, and planning allows your physician to pinpoint the tumor, establish the treatment objectives, and review many treatment options to determine the optimal arrangement and dose of the radiation beams. Respiratory gating then provides the security of protecting healthy structures while targeting the tumor with significantly higher doses of radiation. High doses of radiation ensure the best outcomes: greater control, tumor reduction, and potential cure. Your treatment plan will call for several 20-minute treatments over a period of just weeks. You can return to work or home right after.

St. Vincent's Comprehensive Cancer Center has taken a leadership role by investing in the latest radiation therapy technology. In fact, physicians from leading cancer centers all over the world come in for training. The 24-hour Comprehensive Cancer Center has the most advanced radiation therapy program in the New York metropolitan area.

Proton Therapy

A recent clinical trial at Loma Linda University Medical Center (LLUMC) found that another radiation technique, proton beam radiotherapy, compares favorably with traditional radiation for treatment of early-stage non–small cell lung cancer. With protons, local tumor control was 87 percent, significantly higher than the average 50 percent control rate achieved using traditional radiation.

Published in the fall 1999 issue of the journal *Chest*, these strong clinical results represent encouraging news for lung cancer patients and suggest the possibility of proton therapy as a treatment option.

Dr. David Bush, Department of Radiation Medicine at LLUMC, pointed out that because NSCLC is commonly seen in patients with extensive smoking histories, doctors often must consider their smoking-related illnesses in developing treatment plans. Diseases such as coronary artery disease, peripheral vascular disease, and chronic obstructive pulmonary disease render 15 to 20 percent of them medically inoperable. These patients are potential candidates for proton treatment.

Traditional X-ray (photon) therapy has been used to treat medically inoperable patients, but disease-free survival and local control rates are inferior to those produced by surgery. Proton therapy provides higher radiation, which may enhance survival.

The unique properties of protons provide a distinct physical advantage over conventional X-ray beams. Protons can be controlled and programmed to release their dose in a targeted tumor area. Doses can be increased while reducing the danger to healthy tissue. Pulmonary injury is less significant, and the tumor receives high radiation.

From June 1994 to March 1998, LLUMC treated 37 patients with early-stage NSCLC. Average age was 72, with 27 patients at Stage I, 2 in Stage II, and 8 in Stage IIIA. Trial participants could not have surgery or had refused surgery. Most had significant underlying chronic obstructive pulmonary disease that made surgery too risky.

A future phase of the trial will increase the proton dose delivered and extend this treatment option to patients who have locally advanced lung cancer.

Radiation and Gene Therapy

The response rate in locally advanced lung cancer following radiotherapy given alone is usually less than 18 percent. However, when combined with INGN201, a gene therapy developed by Introgen, radiotherapy provided a threefold increase in response rates, according to new study results.

This lung cancer study was presented at the 2001 ASCO meeting by Stephen Swisher, M.D., of the M. D. Anderson Cancer Center.

Three intratumoral injections of INGN201 were given in conjunction with conventional radiation therapy to 19 people with localized NSCLC who were not eligible for surgery or chemotherapy. Of the 19 patients, 12 had complete or partial responses at the injected site measured three months after completing the treatment. Four patients could not be evaluated. Biopsies confirmed that the tumors were negative for cancer cells.

"This study was designed to efficiently determine how much additional benefit might be afforded to standard radiotherapy when a novel gene therapy was added," said James A. Merritt, M.D., vice president of clinical affairs for Introgen. "We determined that the two treatments can be safely and effectively combined and clinical activity appears to be enhanced. Based on the results, and Introgen's patent that covers combination therapy, this study is a precursor to a Phase III study in which we will further evaluate the approach."

Photodynamic Therapy

QLT PhotoTherapeutics was cleared by the Canadian Health Protection Branch to market its light-activated drug Photofrin as a treatment for certain early- and late-stage lung cancers. Photofrin is already approved in that country for certain esophageal and bladder cancers.

Photodynamic therapy uses lasers to activate light-sensitive drugs. Photodynamic therapy (PDT) with Photofrin can be used to reduce the tumor size and relieve symptoms in patients with completely or partially obstructing endobronchial non–small cell lung cancer. It can also be used for patients who could not qualify for surgery or radiotherapy.

Photofrin, the world's first and only approved photodynamic therapy drug, is now used in the treatment of a number of cancers in 129 cancer centers around the world.

CHEMOTHERAPY

Treatment with chemotherapy does extend the lives of people with advanced lung cancer, according to a national study released at ASCO. More than 1,200 people participated in a Phase III study led by the Eastern Cooperative Oncology Group (ECOG), making it the largest randomized study of lung cancer patients in the United States.

"Survival for lung cancer patients has improved with the use of chemotherapy as a treatment," said lead investigator Dr. Joan H. Schiller, professor at the University of Wisconsin Medical School. "Patients now have a 35 to 40 percent chance of one-year survival, up from 20 to 25 percent five years ago. Lung cancer patients need to be educated about available treatment regiments that may help improve their outcomes."

According to Dr. Robert L. Comis, chair of ECOG, "Only 25 percent of lung cancer patients have historically received chemotherapy treatment despite the fact that research has shown it can prolong their lives. While all four of the chemotherapy regimens studied in the trial are equally effective in terms of prolonging survival, the Taxol plus Paraplatin regimen was shown to be the best tolerated, and maintaining quality of life is a primary objective for patients with advanced disease."

The study was designed to compare three commonly used platinum-based chemotherapy regimens to a reference regimen of cisplatin and Taxol. The experimental regimens in the trial were Taxol plus Paraplatin, Gemzar plus cisplatin, and Taxotere plus cisplatin. Participants all had Stage IIIB or Stage IV NSCLC and had not been previously treated.

There were no significant differences in survival among the three groups of the study when compared with the control group, Taxol and cisplatin. Median survival was eight months. One-year survival was 33 percent and two-year survival was 12 percent. Median time to progression for all groups was 3.6 months.

The regimen of Taxol and Paraplatin showed statistically significant reductions in serious, life-threatening side effects, including hospitalizations. Side effects such as nausea and vomiting were also reduced in the Taxol and Paraplatin arm.

The ECOG was established in 1955 as one of the first cooperative groups launched to perform multicenter cancer clinical trials. Funded primarily by the NCI, the organization has evolved from a five-member consortium of institutions on the East Coast to one of the largest clinical cancer research organizations in the country with more than 5,000 doctors, nurses, pharmacists, statisticians, and clinical research associates from the United States, Canada, and South Africa.

Taxotere

Taking Taxotere on a weekly basis may be preferable to the conventional three-week schedule when it is used as a second-line therapy in patients with NSCLC, according to research reported at the Ninth World Conference on Lung Cancer, held in 2000 in Tokyo.

Of 27 patients treated with weekly Taxotere, 3 had a partial response, 7 had stable disease, and 17 had progressive disease, according to Dr. Rogerio Lilienbaum, of the Mount Sinai Comprehensive Cancer Center in Miami, Florida.

The ongoing Phase II study includes patients with documented recurrent or refractory NSCLC who have received one prior chemotherapy regimen at least one month earlier. Patients with brain metastases are eligible if they are neurologically stable after radiation.

Study participants were treated with Taxotere intravenously over 15 minutes, once a week for six weeks. After a two-week rest period, stable or responding patients continued eight-week courses for as long as they benefited.

Iressa

Iressa, the novel one-a-day anticancer pill, has produced good responses and is well tolerated by patients with advanced NSCLC. Patients were recruited in record numbers for Phase III trials of this drug.

About 10 percent of patients in the Phase I single therapy trials with advanced disease continued on treatment for at least six months. Eight of the patients remained in treatment for one to two years.

Of the 25 patients treated with the combination of Iressa (also known as ZD1839) with this standard chemotherapy regimen, major response or disease stabilization was achieved in 68 percent and one patient had a complete response. The combination of Iressa with carboplatin and paclitaxel is being evaluated as part of the Phase III trial.

"We are encouraged by the safety and activity of the combination in this challenging disease and eagerly await the results of the recently completed Phase II trials. It is hoped that our study will be a prelude to better outcomes for NSCLC patients in the near future," said Dr. Vincent Miller, principal investigator, Memorial Sloan-Kettering Cancer Center in New York.

Final results from a Phase I intermittent dose escalation study of Iressa in Japanese patients with advanced solid tumors including 23 patients with NSCLC were also announced. The patients in this study had been heavily pretreated with up to four chemotherapy regimens. Over 20 percent of the patients with NSCLC showed partial responses to the drug for 1 to 11 months. The drug was well tolerated across a dose escalation range.

WHERE TO FIND INFORMATION ABOUT LUNG CANCER

Alliance for Lung Cancer Advocacy, Support and Education (AL-CASE)
P.O. Box 849
Vancouver, WA 98666
Telephone: 360-696-2436 or 800-298-2436
Web site: www.alcase.org
E-mail: info@alcase.org

This organization provides education, support, advocacy, and an informative newsletter.

American Lung Association (ALA)
1740 Broadway
New York, NY 10019
Telephone: 212-315-8700 or 800-LUNG USA (586-4872)
Web site: www.lungusa.org
E-mail: Info@lungusa.org

The ALA has chapters around the country and they provide a great deal of educational material about lung diseases including lung cancer.

ONGOING CLINICAL TRIALS FOR LUNG CANCER

There are literally hundreds of clinical trials in various stages of development around the world. To list them all here would be misleading because by the time you read this book, some trials may have closed and many others may have opened. Clinical trials have specific eligibility requirements that may eliminate many cancer patients. The few trials listed here are only a sampling of the trials that may be open to you. The best way to locate clinical trials appropriate for your situation is to ask your doctor, check the web sites listed in Chapter 4, and call the biotech companies listed in Appendix C.

1. Clinical trials for patients with chemotherapy-naive Stage IV non–small cell lung cancer to determine the response rate and safety of C225 plus carboplatin and paclitaxel. ImClone, the sponsor, is also running clinical trials for IMC-C225 combined with carboplatin and gemcitabine, and another with docetaxel. This latter is for patients with recurrent or progressive non–small cell lung cancer.

   Contact ImClone in New York at 212-645-1405 or e-mail: clinicaltrials@imclone.com.

2. Aphton is sponsoring clinical trials with Gastrimmune in combination with Taxotere for various cancers including lung, colon, stomach, and prostate.

   Contact Aphton in Miami at 305-374-7615.

3. Cell Genesys is conducting trials of its GVAX vaccine for lung cancer patients. For information call 650-425-4542 or see www.cellgenesys.com.

4. Another vaccine, BLP25, made by the Canadian company, Biomira, was being tested at 10 sites in Canada. Early-phase trials were for 66 people with advanced non–small cell lung cancer who have responded well to standard chemotherapy. Early trials revealed that BLP25 vaccine was well tolerated and capable of triggering a T cell immune response against cancer cells.

5. Agouron Pharmaceuticals is conducting clinical trials of AG3340, an angiogenesis inhibitor, for patients with advanced lung or prostate cancer. Early trials showed the drug to be well tolerated. A randomized trial was expected to be carried out in several sites in North America. The drug was to be administered in tablet form to patients with non–small cell lung cancer in combination with Taxol, Taxotere, and Paraplatin. The primary objective of the trial is to compare time to progression between patients receiving AG3340 or placebo in combination with the chemotherapy drugs.

6. Squalamine, another angiogenesis inhibitor, is being tried in the treatment of non–small cell lung cancer in combination with Taxotere and Paraplatin, the leading cytotoxic chemotherapy regimen for advanced non–small cell lung cancer. Squalamine will be administered intravenously and concurrently with each cycle of chemotherapy. Efficacy will be assessed by the number of patients whose tumors stop growing, along with the number of people who experience tumor shrinkage.

   Trial sites are the M. D. Anderson Cancer Center in Houston (713-792-6161) and the University of Wisconsin Cancer Center in Madison (608-262-5223).

7. In November 2000, a trial of OSI-774, a monoclonal antibody made by OSI Pharmaceuticals in New York, began. This trial used the drug as a single agent and showed that almost half of the 56 patients with advanced, refractory, non–small

cell lung cancer had some disease stabilization after three months on daily oral dosing.

8. The National Cancer Institute and Dow Chemical are conducting trials of a monoclonal antibody known as Mab-CC-49.

CHAPTER 10

▼

BREAKTHROUGH TREATMENTS FOR DIGESTIVE SYSTEM CANCERS

Early detection of colon cancer or colon cancer risk offers physicians and patients a significant advantage in the management and treatment of the disease. Physicians can prescribe subsequent testing of family members, early colon cancer surveillance, detection and removal of polyps, and in some cases prophylactic surgery to help manage the disease. As medicine advances, more drugs are also becoming available to treat colon cancer.

For example, under its license agreement with Genzyme Molecular Oncology, the City of Hope, a nonprofit biomedical research and cancer treatment center in Los Angeles, will perform colon cancer genetic testing services that detect mutations in the MSH2 gene. These mutations, in conjunction with a family history of colon cancer, indicate increased risk for developing hereditary colon cancer.

LabCorp, one of the largest independent clinical diagnostic laboratories in the country, has also licensed rights to the MSH2 gene as well as to the APC gene. Mutations in the APC gene, when accompanied by increased polyps in the patient and a family history of colon cancer, indicate increased risk of developing colon cancer.

According to the American Cancer Society, colon cancer is the leading cause of cancer death among nonsmoking men and women in the United States, with 130,000 new cases and 56,000 deaths projected annually. It is the third leading cause of death by cancer overall in this country. It is now believed by medical scientists that about 25 percent of colon cancer cases are triggered by a genetic predisposition to the disease.

Surgery is the primary treatment method for colorectal cancer. This means removing the cancerous areas and some surrounding normal tissue. Nearby lymph nodes are also removed. After surgery the continuity of the bowel is restored by joining the healthy ends, a procedure called anastomosis. Sometimes a temporary colostomy is performed. A colostomy is a procedure that attaches part of the colon to a bag outside the body to collect waste matter. This gives the body time to heal and is "reversed" when the colon is able to work normally again. A colonoscopy is an endoscopic procedure used to examine—and photograph—the inside of the entire colon. At the time of the exam, if a polyp is seen in the colon, it can be removed with a tiny instrument inserted through the endoscopic tube. Very early colon cancers often can be removed by colonoscopy.

Treatment of rectal cancer often combines surgery with chemotherapy and radiation. Sometimes chemotherapy is given before surgery to shrink tumors. After surgery, chemotherapy may be used as a palliative measure if surgery did not completely remove the tumor and the disease has spread. The drugs commonly used are a combination of 5-fluorouracil (5-FU) with levamisole or leucovorin. More recently, that regimen is followed with irinotecan (see below).

GENETICS OF COLON CANCER

In the latest of a series of discoveries about colon cancer genes, researchers at the Johns Hopkins Oncology Center and the Howard Hughes Medical Institute discovered a connection between two of them—APC and c-MYC—that conspires to initiate almost all colon cancers. All of us carry the c-MYC oncogene, but it remains under control in the colon until awakened by the failure of the tumor suppressor gene.

A cancer is like a car with the accelerator pushed to the floor and failing brakes. In this case, c-MYC is the accelerator and APC is the failed brakes. When suppressor genes, like APC, malfunction either through heredity or as a result of exposure to carcinogens, cells get signals to continue multiplying until they are out of control. Now we know that in colon cancer a mutated APC gene signals ineffectively to c-MYC.

Johns Hopkins scientists Bert Vogelstein, M.D., and Kenneth W. Kinzler, Ph.D., have found that the mutated APC gene controls the expression of c-MYC activation. APC was first identified and linked to colon cancer in 1991 by research teams including those led by Vogelstein and Kinzler.

The new findings about the APC pathway and how it functions suggest potential new drug strategies that could prevent colon cancer by blocking the signal that activates c-MYC. Just eight years ago, we didn't even know about APC mutations. Now we know that this type of mutation is one of the earliest genetic changes in most colon cancers, and we know what it does to c-MYC. It's like a jigsaw puzzle. We have identified individual pieces of the cancer puzzle, and now we can begin to put them together to see the whole picture of how they work together to cause cancer.

MONOCLONAL ANTIBODIES FOR COLON CANCER

ImClone Systems' C225 clinical trials were the subject of a CBS-TV *60 Minutes* program in May 2001 over the way patients with advanced colorectal cancer are selected for the trials. Many who qualified were unable to get the drug through the company's compassionate use mechanism.

Studies show that when C225, a monoclonal antibody, is combined with irinotecan, a chemotherapy agent, tumors shrink and the progress of the disease slows down. In 22.5 percent of patients tumors shrank. This exceeds the 15 percent response rate needed for the drug to win FDA approval, according to ImClone's president, Dr. Samuel Waskal. Dr. Leonard Saltz of Memorial Sloan-Kettering Cancer Center, who led the trials, stressed that it is not a cure but that patients who respond will live longer.

C225 is designed to target and block the epidermal growth factor receptor (EGFR), a protein that is expressed on the surface of cancer cells. Most cases of metastatic colorectal carcinoma are positive for EGFR expression. Normal cells may have 10,000 copies of this receptor, but cancer cells have more than a million.

As many as 70 to 80 percent of colon cancers—as well as prostate, lung, and head and neck cancers—may have this excess EGFR. The receptor is also called Her1 and is in the same family as Her2, the protein that is blocked by Herceptin, a breast cancer drug (see page 59).

C225 is one of two types of EGFR-blocking drugs, which are monoclonal antibodies (MABs). There are others in early stages of development. MABs are engineered versions of the proteins the body uses to fight off germs. They are given intravenously and they bind to the receptors protruding from the tumor cell surface, preventing the intended growth factor from binding. The most common side effect is an acnelike rash that goes away when treatment stops.

Treatment with C225 and irinotecan may represent a promising step in treatment for colorectal carcinoma patients who have gone through standard therapy. Samuel Waskal, Ph.D., president of ImClone, said, "We have made great progress here at ImClone at moving to a new therapy for colon cancer." The data are being prepared as quickly as possible for review by the FDA.

Other cancer-fighting therapies in development include IMC-1C11, designed to inhibit tumor angiogenesis by blocking the vascular endothelial growth factor (VEGF) from binding to the VEGF receptor, also known as the KDR receptor. It is being tested in a Phase I study. BEC2 is a vaccine designed to prevent or delay the recurrence of certain types of tumors by mimicking the GD3 tumor antigen, a molecule found on the surface of several types of cancer cells. By mimicking this antigen, BEC2 appears to stimulate a stronger immune response to cells expressing natural GD3. BEC2 is in Phase III trials.

ImClone is developing a next generation of cancer treatments, that is, products that can be used directly as cancer therapeutics or indirectly as cancer vaccines. Cancer therapeutics interrupt the molecular basis of tumor development and survival. ImClone focuses on the differences between normal cells and developing tumor cells, and on the ways tumor cells are able to circumvent the normal regulatory mechanisms or "biologic checkpoints" that control cell division and cell proliferation. Cancer vaccines, on the other hand, stimulate the body's immune system to produce an antitumor response. The clinical affairs department is responsible for these trials and can be reached at clinicaltrials@imclone.com.

VACCINES FOR COLON CANCER

In 2000, the Cancer Research Institute started a groundbreaking program of funding for research called the Colon Cancer Collaborative. This program provides money and encourages collaboration among teams of researchers around the world with a common goal. The institute can quickly mobilize new breakthroughs for colon cancer.

The collaborative began from one woman's personal experience. Dr. Christa Maar of the Hubert Burda Foundation for Cancer Research in Munich, Germany, had a 34-year-old son who was diagnosed with advanced colon cancer. This set her on a mission to find out what was going on in current colon cancer research. She found cancer centers all over the world involved in their own—and different—treatment methods. Eventually, Dr. Maar contributed $3 million to establish the collaborative for developing effective immunological strategies to diagnose, treat, and prevent colon cancer.

The benefits became clear when Dr. Haruo Ohtani, a Japanese pathologist, observed that colon cancer patients whose tumors are infiltrated by lymphocytes have a better prognosis than patients with tumors without such lymphocyte invasion. This led him to analyze the antibody response of patients with colon cancer to their own cancer cells and to develop a more comprehensive picture of the immune system response to colon cancer. When colon cancer antigens are defined, effective vaccines can be developed.

Theratope

Biomira, a Canadian biotech company, reported in 2001 that their Phase II clinical trial of Theratope vaccine suggests that people with metastatic colorectal cancer live longer. The study of 45 patients was conducted at the University of Nebraska. Ten of the patients had rectal cancer and 35 had colon cancer. Dr. Margaret Tempero, deputy director of the University of California at San Francisco Comprehensive Cancer Center, conducted the study.

Theratope is designed to stimulate the body's immune system to mount a response against the cancer cells. The vaccine is generally well tolerated and may be suitable for other cancers, too.

Gastrimmune

The Aphton Corporation of Miami is using its innovative vaccinelike technology for neutralizing hormones that participate in the gastrointestinal system. The company believes that an immunochemotherapy regimen that includes Gastrimmune can extend patient survival without adding toxicity. Gastrimmune blocks the action of the gastrin 17 hormone.

Gastrimmune is the lead product in an advanced clinical trials program for treatment of colorectal and stomach cancer. Forty patients with colorectal cancer that had spread to distant organs were treated with Gastrimmune. The study was carried out at the Queen's Medical Center, University of Nottingham in England.

The patients immunized with Gastrimmune survived 338 days compared to 184 days for those who did not receive the vaccine. "These clinical results in human patients were very dramatic and give hope where none has been possible before," said Dov Michaeli, M.D., Ph.D., Aphton's chief medical officer. "Perhaps the most impressive aspect of these results is that, to my knowledge, no drug has shown a survival extension for end-stage colorectal cancer which even remotely approaches that of Gastrimmune."

Owing to its impact on life-threatening cancers, Gastrimmune should now be on a fast track for approval early in the 21st century. Aphton is beginning a clinical trial with patients who have failed the approved chemotherapy regimen of 5-FU and irinotecan for Dukes' D stage colorectal cancer. Patients will be treated with a combination regimen of Aphton's anti-G17 immunogen and irinotecan. The company plans to file for a fast-track marketing approval when enough terminal patients respond to treatment.

Although the price of the drug has been estimated at about $10,000 per patient, one $5,000 injection followed by semiannual booster shots also at $5,000, this is far cheaper than today's radiation or chemotherapy and intensive care hospitalization treatments.

CHEMOTHERAPY FOR COLON CANCER

Irinotecan

Irinotecan is the first new agent approved for colon cancer in almost 40 years. In 1995 in Japan and Europe, irinotecan (CPT-11) was licensed for advanced colorectal cancers previously treated with 5-FU, a standard chemotherapy. In June 1996, after review of three Phase II trials, the FDA approved irinotecan for patients with metastatic colorectal carcinoma whose disease has recurred or progressed following 5-FU-based chemotherapy. In the United States, irinotecan is available from the Pharmacia & Upjohn Company as Camptosar.

Irinotecan is a topoisomerase I inhibitor, a new class of chemotherapeutic agents with a unique mechanism of action. Scientists searching for a natural source of steroids discovered the parent compound camptothecin in the 1960s. This compound interferes with DNA synthesis and therefore results in tumor cell death.

Three main topoisomerase I inhibitors are currently in clinical trials with 304 patients: topotecan (for ovarian cancer), 9-aminocamptothecin, and irinotecan. Although topotecan has shown activity in many solid tumors, it has not yet demonstrated clinical effectiveness in colon cancers. Aminocamptothecin is in an early stage of clinical development. Preclinical data show it to be effective in colorectal cancers, but this has yet to be demonstrated in the laboratory.

All patients had measurable metastatic colorectal cancer that was resistant to one fluorouracil-containing regimen, but were otherwise in good condition. The average time to response was 2.7 months, with the majority of responses occurring after the first two courses of therapy. The median duration of response was approximately 6 months, with a median survival duration of 9 months.

Xeloda

The FDA has approved Xeloda, the first oral chemotherapy for the treatment of metastatic colorectal cancer. Xeloda works by activating enzymes to interact with the cancer-fighting drug 5-FU. The human body produces the enzyme thymidine phosphorylase, which converts Xeloda into 5-FU.

"Because Xeloda is a pill, it allows people with colorectal cancer the flexibility of taking their medication on the go without interrupting work or other activities," said John Marshall, M.D., director of the developmental therapeutics program at the Lombardi Cancer Center at Georgetown University Medical Center.

Xeloda, made by Roche, is only the second new treatment for colorectal cancer approved in the United States in the past 40 years. Xeloda is indicated as first-line treatment for those with metastatic colorectal cancer when treatment with fluoropyrimidine therapy alone is preferred. Xeloda is covered by Medicare.

The FDA decision was based on the results of two multinational Phase III clinical trials that revealed that the drug shrinks tumors better than the standard-of-care intravenous 5-FU and leucovorin, known as the Mayo Regimen. Xeloda requires only two daily pills compared to the more complex intravenous regimen.

PREVENTION STRATEGY FOR COLON CANCER

In the 1970s, Dr. William Waddell of the University of Colorado Health Sciences Center in Denver treated a patient with familial adenomatous polyposis, the rare hereditary type of colon cancer. Her colon had been removed when she was 23 to prevent her getting the disease. But at 31 she developed noncancerous scarlike tumors in her abdomen and polyps were growing in her rectum. Dr. Waddell prescribed indomethacin, an anti-inflammatory drug that often makes such tumors shrink. When the drug upset her stomach after years of treatment, Dr. Waddell added another anti-inflammatory, sulindac. To his surprise the tumors disappeared. Over the years, Dr. Waddell prescribed the drug to similar patients, with some success. He published papers in medical journals but few of his peers believed him. Finally, it got national attention in 1993 when others tested it and the *New England Journal of Medicine* published one study.

Now scientists are looking at these aspirinlike drugs used to treat arthritis as a way to prevent colon cancer. This discovery was made accidentally, but with the development of Celebrex at Searle, research is continuing. It is aimed at a large group of arthritis sufferers who needed anti-inflammatory drugs without the gastrointestinal side effects. Cox-2 is an enzyme involved in inflammation. Until recently, the only drugs that blocked it had a troublesome side effect, such as gastrointestinal bleeding. New cox-2 inhibitors were developed to prevent this problem, so people with arthritis and other inflammatory conditions would be able to take drugs for pain relief.

The Searle-NCI study found that patients who took Celebrex had a 28 percent reduction in the number of polyps, compared to a 5 percent reduction in those taking a placebo. The study included 83 patients for six months. The FDA approved the drug late in 2000 for patients with familial adenopolyposis (FAP).

NCI and Searle are conducting studies of thousands of Americans to find out if a drug like Celebrex can prevent cancer. Merck is starting a similar study on its own. Previous animal and lab studies lend support to the idea.

CHEMOTHERAPY FOR STOMACH CANCER

A form of stomach cancer called gastrointestinal stromal tumors (GISTs) is not as rare as once thought, according to scientists gathered in 2001 at the American Society of Clinical Oncologists (ASCO). There are about 5,000 to 10,000 cases diagnosed in the United States each year. GIST is resistant to most therapies. However, Gleevec, recently approved for treatment of a type of leukemia, may be effective for this disease.

There was an 89 percent improvement rate in the first test of this drug in solid tumors. Two studies demonstrate a remarkable response to a new signal transduction inhibitor (STI) in solid tumors. Both studies looked at Gleevec, then known as STI-571, in patients with advanced GISTs, according to researchers at Oregon Health Sciences University. In the Phase II clinical trial of 139 patients, fewer than 1 percent had responded to previous therapies, but 68 patients had a partial response and 54 had stable disease.

"These results are very exciting and demonstrate the value of therapy that is molecularly targeted at what makes a cell cancerous," said the lead author, Charles Blanke, M.D., an oncologist at Oregon Health Sciences University. "For the first time, STI-571 is showing tremendous benefit in a solid tumor." STIs interfere with the enzymes that trigger tumor cell growth. In GIST, Gleevec blocks the growth signal of C-KIT, a gene that is overexpressed and promotes cell proliferation.

At least one person in New York has already been released from a hospice because the cancer shrank. Before that, Gleevec benefits in GIST came from the case of a woman in Finland who has now been free of the disease for more than a year. In trials, Gleevec produced complete remissions in more than 180 GIST patients in the United States and Europe.

Of the 86 patients who took the drug for three or more months in a study with Dr. Charles Blanke, 59 percent went into remission. The average follow-up is four and a half months, but nobody who achieved remission and is still taking the drug has relapsed. What makes this so exciting is that most GISTs progress within six months, and they have always been resistant to chemotherapy and radiation.

Dr. Larry Norton of Memorial Sloan-Kettering Cancer Center told the *New York Times*, "All of a sudden, almost miraculously, we have a drug that works in most cases for one of the hardest cancers to treat and might even be a cure." This could be like insulin for a diabetic, something you take for the rest of your life. Future trials will bring the answer.

GIST strikes as many people as the better-known Hodgkin's disease. GIST tumors develop in the connective tissue—stroma—of the intestines and can develop anywhere in the digestive system from the esophagus to the colon. Tumors can cause pain, weight loss, and such severe bloating as to make one appear pregnant.

However, some patients did not achieve remission with the drug, and scientists still don't know if GIST cells might become resistant to Gleevec. The drug also has life-threatening side effects, such as bleeding in one of four patients. Less serious are nausea, skin rash, and swelling of the legs. Experts still don't know how long someone can take the drug or if they can ever stop. Gleevec can cost up to $2,400 a month.

While the FDA has approved Gleevec only for leukemia, it can be prescribed by your doctor for other conditions. This practice is known as off-label use. Dr. Blanke and his collaborator in Belgium, Dr. Allan T. vanOosterom of the University of Leuven, did not think that was a good idea yet.

Because patients have been demanding Gleevec, the NCI has started a larger clinical trial now being conducted at scores of hospitals around the country.

Gleevec is made by Novartis. It is like a guided missile, killing only cancer cells and sparing healthy ones. That it is so effective in two completely different cancers has surprised researchers who have long been bragging about the potential of molecularly targeted drugs.

EXPERIMENTAL TREATMENTS FOR ESOPHAGEAL CANCER

Stomach cancer is less common in the United States today than it was 70 years ago, but esophageal cancer is on the rise. Research is under way to diagnose this cancer sooner, in order to repair the DNA. Immunotherapy is currently in clinical trials, using monoclonal antibodies to seek out cancer cells with excess proteins like CEA (carcinoembryonic antigen) or the HER2 oncogene.

A short course of chemotherapy before surgery is helping patients live longer, according to a British study reported in May 2001. And while there are no long-term results yet, if you have this cancer, you should urge your doctor to consider this treatment.

According to the National Institutes of Health, photodynamic therapy (PDT), a type of laser therapy, is being used to relieve symptoms of esophageal cancer such as difficulty in swallowing. The patient takes drugs that are absorbed by the cancer cells. When exposed to a special light, the drugs become active and destroy the cancer cells.

CHEMOTHERAPY FOR PANCREATIC CANCER

Don, 51, was given four months to live when doctors found a tumor the size of a tennis ball in his pancreas. This lethal cancer had killed actors Michael Landon and Marcello Mastroianni in addition to thousands of less well-known patients. Fortunately for Don, he learned that the Stehlin Foundation for Cancer Research in Houston was beginning human testing on an extraordinary cancer-fighting compound we now call Rubitecan. Six weeks after he started taking Rubitecan, Don's deadly tumor had shrunk to the size of a golf ball. Today he tells everyone who will listen, "All that's left of that tumor is some scar tissue. It's gone. Thank God. Four months have turned into four years now. And I feel great. It's really hard to believe I came so close to death."

Until recently few people had hope of surviving this insidious cancer. It killed Michael Landon at a young age, and it kills 28,000 other Americans every year. Now, SuperGen's Rubitecan has lengthened the lives of at least that many people with pancreatic cancer, and hundreds of thousands more with other types of cancer, according to Joseph Rubinfeld, Ph.D., chairman and CEO of SuperGen.

A Phase II study showed that treatment with SuperGen's oral 9-nitrocamptothecin (9NC, RFS 2000) either shrank pancreatic tumors or stabilized the disease in 63 percent of patients with advanced disease. The median survival time among patients who responded to treatment was 18.6 months, which is the longest survival time ever reported among advanced pancreatic cancer patients.

The cause of pancreatic cancer is unknown, but age and smoking are risk factors—smoking doubles the risk. There is also a possible link with chronic pancreatitis, diabetes, or cirrhosis. The only hereditary factor may be a family predisposition to diabetes. Diabetes is found in about 20 to 40 percent of all cases, most often in women. Pancreatic cancer rates are higher in countries with a diet high in fat. As with colon and stomach cancers, the survival rate for pancreatic cancer is low because there are no symptoms of the disease until it is in the advanced stages and has metastasized.

Surgery, radiation therapy, and chemotherapy can extend survival or relieve symptoms but are unlikely to provide a cure. Gemcitabine is the chemotherapy drug of choice, but in only about 25 percent of patients is there a prolonging of life or an improvement in symptoms with its use.

WHERE TO FIND INFORMATION ABOUT DIGESTIVE SYSTEM CANCERS

Colon Cancer Alliance
175 Ninth Avenue
New York, NY 10011
Telephone: 212-627-7451
Web site: www.ccalliance.org

This organization provides information and support programs. It also has links to clinical trials all over the world for colon cancer.

Colorectal Cancer Network
P.O. Box 182
Kensington, MD 20895-0182
Telephone: 301-879-1500
Web site: www.colorectal-cancer.net
E-mail: ccnetwork@colorectal-cancer.net
This organization provides information and support programs. It also has links to clinical trials all over the world for colon cancer.

United Ostomy Association, Inc.
Suite 200
19772 MacArthur Boulevard
Irvine, CA 92612-2405
Telephone: 949-660-8624 or 800-826-0826
Web site: www.uoa.org
E-mail: uoa@deltanet.com
This organization provides information and support programs. It also has links to clinical trials all over the world for colon cancer.

ONGOING CLINICAL TRIALS FOR DIGESTIVE SYSTEM CANCERS

There are literally hundreds of clinical trials in various stages of development around the world. To list them all here would be misleading because by the time you read this book, some trials may have closed and many others may have opened. Clinical trials have specific eligibility requirements that may eliminate many cancer patients. The few trials listed here are only a sampling of the trials that may be open to you. The best way to locate clinical trials appropriate for your situation is to ask your doctor, check the web sites listed in Chapter 4, and call the biotech companies listed in Appendix C.

Ongoing Clinical Trials for Colon Cancer

1. A Phase I trial to study the effectiveness of a combination chemotherapy and radiation after surgery. Patients will receive uracil, tegafur, and leucovorin orally three times a day for four weeks followed by one week without treatment; then radiation therapy once a day plus chemotherapy for four more weeks.

   Contact Bruce David Minsky at Memorial Sloan-Kettering Cancer Center in New York at 212-639-6817.

2. A Phase I trial to study the effectiveness of a vaccine containing mutated Ras peptides and an immune adjuvant in treating patients who have colon, pancreatic, or lung cancer. Patients will receive an injection of the peptide once a month for at least three months. You must be at least 19 and have no central nervous system metastasis. Also, it must be at least four weeks since previous therapy.

   Contact Samir N. Khleif, chair, Center for Cancer Research, Bethesda, MD, 301-496-0901.

3. A Phase I trial of LMB-9 Immunotoxin in patients with advanced colon cancer. (This is also enrolling patients with breast, non–small cell lung, bladder, pancreas, and ovarian cancer.)

   Contact: NCI sponsored. Judith E. Karp, chair, Marlene and Steward Greenebaum Cancer Center, University of Maryland, 410-328-7394.

4. Phase I/II study of adjuvant autologous tumor cell vaccine in patients with completely resected Stage II or III colon cancer. Vaccines made from the patient's own white blood cells will be used to build an immune response. The vaccine therapy will be combined with leucovorin and fluorouracil to treat patients who have had surgery to completely remove the colon cancer and who show no metastasis.

   Contact William Gannon at the Intracel Corporation at 301-258-5200. Other contacts include Lee E. Smith at the Washington Hospital Center in DC at 202-877-8484; Armondo

Sardi at St. Agnes Healthcare in Baltimore, 410-368-2702; Linda L. Lapos, Lehigh Valley Hospital in Allentown, PA, 610-402-1095; Thomas Patrick Wright at Inova Fairfax Hospital in Virginia at 703-560-7788.

5. A Phase I/II study of monoclonal antibody 105AD7 anti-idiotype vaccine and ONYCR1, ONYCR2, and ONYCR3 allogeneic adenocarcinoma cell–based vaccines in patients with locally advanced or metastatic cancer of the colon or rectum. Some patients will receive injections of monoclonal antibodies alone; others will receive vaccine therapy alone. A third group will receive monoclonal antibodies and chemotherapy combined. This is an NCI-sponsored trial with Onyvax.

Contact Fiona Lofts at Onyvax Limited at St. George's Hospital in London, England, at 020-8725-0231.

6. Phase I/II study of Ras peptide cancer vaccine with or without interleukin-2 in HLA A2.1 positive patients with locally advanced or metastatic colon or rectal cancer.

Contact John Edward Janik at Vanderbilt-Ingram Cancer Center in Nashville at 301-402-2913, or Jay A. Berzofsky at the Center for Cancer Research, Metabolism Branch, Bethesda, MD, at 301-496-6874.

7. Phase I/II trial of SU5416 and irinotecan in patients with advanced colon cancer. Patients must have measurable disease but no previous treatment with these two drugs. It must be at least four weeks since radiation or surgery and there must be no central nervous system metastasis.

Contact James L. Abbruzzese of the M. D. Anderson Cancer Center at the University of Texas at 713-792-2828.

Ongoing Clinical Trials for Stomach or Esophageal Cancer

1. A Phase I trial to study the effectiveness of decitabine-mediated induction of tumor antigen and tumor suppressor gene expression in patients with inoperable esophageal or lung cancer or malignant pleural mesothelioma.

Contact David Schrump at the Center for Cancer Research, surgery branch, in Bethesda, MD, at 301-496-2127.

2. A randomized Phase II trial using a vaccine to build an immune response to kill tumor cells in the gastrointestinal tract.

Contact Robert P. Whitehead at the University of Texas Medical Branch at 409-772-1164.

Ongoing Clinical Trials for Pancreatic Cancer

1. Rubitecan (RFS2000) is currently an investigational drug from SuperGen that is being evaluated for treatment of pancreatic cancer in three large-scale randomized multicenter studies involving more than 1,800 patients from about 200 clinical study sites in North America and Europe. The drug is also under evaluation for treatment of a wide variety of other tumor types (such as breast, ovarian, lung, bladder, and prostate cancer) in more than 30 clinical studies in the United States and Europe.

Contact the SuperGen clinical hot line at 925-327-0200, extension 320.

2. A Phase I trial to study the effectiveness of vaccines made from mutated Ras peptides to build an immune response to fight pancreatic cancer. (It is also being studied in lung and colon cancer.) You must be at least 19 years old and have no central nervous system metastasis. Also, it must be at least four weeks since you had any other type of treatment. You will receive an injection of the peptide once a month for at least three months.

Contact Samir N. Khleif at the Center for Cancer Research, Bethesda, MD, at 301-496-0901.

3. A phase II study of the effectiveness of gemcitabine and radiotherapy in patients who have had pancreatic surgery. You must be at least 19 and have had no previous chemotherapy or radiation for pancreatic cancer. And no more than two months has gone by since surgery to remove your tumor. You

will be given infusions of gemcitabine twice a week for five weeks. At the same time, you will receive radiation therapy.

Contact Arthur William Blackstock at the Comprehensive Cancer Center of Wake Forest University Baptist Medical Center, Winston-Salem, NC, at 336-716-4668.

4. A Phase II trial for gemcitabine and trastuzumab (monoclonal antibody: Herceptin) in patients with an overexpression of HER2/neu, who have not been treated with Herceptin before. Combining this with conventional chemotherapy may be more effective in treating this cancer.

Contact Howard Safran of the Center for Cancer Research in Bethesda, MD, at 401-793-7151.

CHAPTER 11

▼

BREAKTHROUGH TREATMENTS FOR LEUKEMIA, LYMPHOMA, AND MULTIPLE MYELOMA

It's not every day or every new drug that gets the universal media fanfare that came with the FDA approval in May 2001 for Gleevec, a biotech drug that showed remarkable remission rates for a type of leukemia. Tommy G. Thompson, the U.S. secretary of health and human services, announced the speedy approval at a national press conference along with Dr. Richard Klausner, director of the National Cancer Institute, and Dr. Daniel Vasella, chairman and CEO of Novartis, the company that developed the drug.

The FDA approved the drug after only a two-and-a-half month review of the clinical data—an all-time record for a cancer drug—in an effort to highlight the hopes for the new drug and the government's role in bringing it to market. It usually takes six months to approve drugs accepted for priority review.

CHEMOTHERAPY FOR LEUKEMIA

Gleevec for Chronic Myelogenous Leukemia

Gleevec is designed just to kill leukemia cells. It's a whole different approach. We know the cause of cancer, at least in general. The mutation of certain genes is believed to be the start of malignant growth in cells. Of the 30,000 human genes that are now known, only 300 or 400 are important for cancer. If those genes are not working, the cell either dies or becomes malignant. If a drug can knock out one or two of these target genes, the cancer can be stopped.

It took 16 years to perfect Gleevec, and according to Dr. Klausner, it is the "first molecularly targeted drug." The FDA granted swift approval to Gleevec for chronic myelogenous leukemia (CML), one of the four main types of leukemia, which affects about 20 percent of leukemia patients. The pace of the project speeded up as investigators found that the drug was well tolerated in over 1,000 patients around the world. When you have the right target with the right disease, there is a much quicker time to market.

Not only was it the first molecular targeting drug to reach approval, but patients themselves are the story behind this remarkably speedy approval. They pressured their doctors, the drug companies, and the government, demanding that the drug be made available because it was so effective and gave them none of the debilitating side effects of chemotherapy.

The results of Gleevec were immediate and striking. In one trial of 54 patients, the drug caused blood counts to revert to normal in 90 percent of the cases and cancerous cells to disappear altogether in 13 percent. The side effects were minimal.

While chemotherapy and other forms of cancer therapy harm all dividing cells, Gleevec hits the cancer cells' key enzymes specifically, thus avoiding the overwhelming side effects. It is the first in a new class of drugs that disrupt specific signaling proteins that are liable to run amok in cancer and cause the cell to divide incessantly.

Dr. Brian Drucker, of the Oregon Health Sciences University, said that while a third of these patients are candidates for bone marrow transplants, the rest have to rely on interferon. He said that after ten months of taking medication, there is still evidence of the disease in their bone marrow.

CML is characterized by a chromosomal abnormality—the so-called Philadelphia chromosome. It can be controlled but not cured with chemotherapy. Interferon has also been used alone or in combination with chemotherapy. Bone marrow transplantation with a related or unrelated donor has cured many younger patients.

The word *leukemia* means "white blood." The bone marrow produces a large number of abnormal white blood cells; some people have so many white blood cells that the blood has a whitish cast. Leukemia interferes with the body's ability to fight infection, and it begins with one or a few white blood cells that have a lost or damaged DNA sequence. These cells do not mature but rather stay in an immature, or blast, state. They are still capable of multiplying, however. Rather than mature and die like normal cells, they collect and interfere with body functions.

Gleevec gives hope to the 5,000 people in North America who have CML. "We are really witnessing an enormous payoff of years of investment in cancer research," said William Hait, M.D., director of the Cancer Institute of New Jersey at New Brunswick.

Novartis, the international pharmaceutical company based in Switzerland, has initiated a 20-center international study of Gleevec for CML patients and is close to meeting a recruitment goal of up to 1,000 patients.

Because of the short-term nature of the clinical tests for Gleevec, researchers warn that with long-term use, side effects or serious resistance to the drug could develop. The average survival time for someone with myelogenous leukemia is six years, and clinical trials of Gleevec only started in June 1998.

Other than CML, Gleevec seems to be effective in a gastrointestinal stromal tumor or GIST, which is usually incurable if surgery fails. (See Chapter 10 for more about Gleevec and GIST.) Doctors are suggesting that the Novartis drug, which produced a 100 percent remission rate in advanced leukemia in the Phase I trials, may also be effective against brain and lung cancers.

Novartis said Gleevec would cost $2,000 to $2,400 a month. However, the company said it would supply the drug for less to people not covered by medical insurance. You can get the drug free if you earn less than $43,000 a year, and at a discount if you earn up to $200,000 a year. Dr. Vasella said the price of Gleevec compares to current therapy, but that it will provide much more value to patients because it is more effective and better tolerated.

The medical and scientific community all accept that in time the cancer treatment will be designed at the molecular level. The more that you can strike at cancer itself, and disrupt the cancer-specific signaling machinery, the less toxic and harmful the cancer treatment will be. We are embarking on a science-intensive form of cancer treatment. Now the scientific tools are there. We can design drugs that intervene at a specific place in the cancer process.

The radical change in therapy that is the result of molecular targeting was described by Dr. David Scheinberg, chief of leukemia services at Memorial Sloan-Kettering Cancer Center in New York. He said that now there are many therapies for leukemia and they can be targeted to a specific patient and his disease. It's now more important than ever to seek out the very best cancer care available. At Memorial Sloan-Kettering they are now able to treat leukemia by tailoring the therapy to each patient's disease. This means that, rather than just getting the standard treatment for leukemia, each patient has his own targeted therapy, which gives him a much better chance for survival and remission than in years past.

Mylotarg for Acute Myelogenous Leukemia

In May 2000, a year before the Gleevec approval, the FDA approved Mylotarg, the first targeted chemotherapy agent using monoclonal antibody technology for leukemia. Marketed by Wyeth-Ayerst Laboratories in Madison, New Jersey, Mylotarg also got accelerated approval—although not as swiftly as Gleevec—for the treatment of patients 60 and older with CD33-positive acute myelogenous leukemia (AML) who are not considered candidates for cytotoxic chemotherapy and whose cancer has recurred. However, without long-term studies, the safety of Mylotarg in AML patients has not been established.

AML is the most common type of acute leukemia in adults. The American Cancer Society has estimated that 9,700 new cases of AML will occur in the United States each year. More than three-fourths of patients with AML are over the age of 60, and 75 percent of patients with AML ultimately relapse.

The effectiveness of Mylotarg is based solely on patient response rates. In three multinational Phase II trials, involving 142 patients, Mylotarg as a single agent produced a 26 percent overall remission rate in these patients. Overall survival for the patients was 5.9 months.

Mylotarg is a humanized antibody linked with a potent antitumor antibiotic called calicheamicin, a bacterium found in a caliche clay soil sample from Texas. The antibody portion of Mylotarg binds specifically to the CD33 antigen, a protein commonly expressed by myeloid leukemic cells. Such precise targeting means an anticancer agent might search out and destroy only cancer cells while sparing normal cells and tissue. In addition, targeting only cancer cells could mean doctors could use higher doses of conventional chemotherapy drugs that would otherwise be too toxic to administer.

Mylotarg's discovery and development began with the discovery of a soil organism. Wyeth-Ayerst had a program that screened soil organisms from around the world for possible new drug products. Employees were asked to bring back soil samples from wherever they traveled. In 1981, one returned with a sample of caliche clay collected near Kerrville, Texas. The clay contained an organism that produced a molecule called calicheamicin gamma. Researchers isolated this as a white powder and found it was a cell-killing antibiotic. They also discovered it was as much as 10,000 times more toxic to cells than traditional anticancer drugs.

Because it is so deadly to cells, calicheamicin cannot be infused directly into humans, as chemotherapy is normally delivered. So researchers needed to find a way to deliver the drug very selectively to the cells. They needed an antigen that was unique to the surface of the cancer cell. If they could identify an antigen, then a monoclonal antibody could be developed to bind to that antigen and deliver a molecule of calicheamicin right to the cell.

The CD33 was discovered by Dr. Irwin Bernstein of the Fred Hutchinson Cancer Research Center in Seattle, whose work focused on antigens related to AML. He suggested the company use one he had discovered in mice, which he was using to study AML. The CD33 antibody proved to be the one they needed. It appears on the AML cells in most patients with the disease. The antibody extends the life of the drug, so calicheamicin can circulate in the blood for days. And once it locks with the CD33 antigen, it rapidly escorts the drug inside the cell.

Successful human trials, led by Dr. Eric Sievers at the Fred Hutchinson Cancer Research Center, began in May 1995, and eventually involved many international sites. These clinical studies proved the drug reasonably safe and moderately effective. This led to the FDA approval in 2000 of Mylotarg for the treatment of certain leukemia patients.

Chemotherapy can bring about a cure in 25 to 30 percent of children and young adults with AML. One or two cycles of chemotherapy are given to achieve remission. Further cycles are given to consolidate remission. Other new treatments under evaluation are interleukin-2 and modifiers of drug resistance. For younger patients with a suitable sibling donor, bone marrow transplantation in the first remission may be the best chance for a cure. The use of the patient's own bone marrow for transplantation is also a possibility.

"We anticipate Mylotarg being an important treatment option for older patients with relapsed CD33-positive AML who frequently cannot tolerate conventional combination chemotherapy," said L. Patrick Gage, Ph.D., president of Wyeth-Ayerst Research. "Mylotarg can be administered in outpatient settings. This may be desirable to many patients," Dr. Gage added.

Arsenic for Acute Promyelocytic Leukemia

An old folk remedy from rural China is proving to be a cure for an uncommon but particularly devastating form of leukemia. In the United States, acute promyelocytic leukemia (APL) represents 10 to 15 percent of the more than 10,000 patients who are diagnosed with acute myelogenous leukemia each year. Now, at Dana-

Farber, Memorial Sloan-Kettering, and other cancer centers, this Chinese treatment is routinely used, and it is the subject of several trials involving a dozen other cancers, as well. Arsenic trioxide (Trisenox) was approved by the FDA for patients with APL in September of 2000.

Known as Drug 731, it has not had a glamorous development as the biotech drugs have. It is based on an old theory of traditional Chinese medicine of giving poison to cure poison. It was discovered in a mud hut in China: a powdery home brew of types of ground rock and the venom of a local toad. People drank it or rubbed it on their skin. Sometimes doctors wrapped it in newspapers and placed it on infected wounds. But the dosage, naturally, must remain small, so the road to recovery is a long one.

Clinical trials with Trisenox showed that a good number of those patients who had multiple relapses were able to achieve a complete remission, or a disappearance of all visible leukemia cells. The majority of those who achieved complete remission were still disease free after 16 months.

A trial with 40 patients with relapsed APL unresponsive to standard therapies was conducted at Memorial Sloan-Kettering Cancer Center by Dr. Steven Soignet, a physician on the developmental chemotherapy service, and also in the Department of Medicine, Cornell University Medical Center, both in New York City. Seventy percent had a complete remission, and the genetic abnormality associated with APL was eradicated in the majority of patients. Complete remission was achieved on average within two months after starting treatment with Trisenox.

Though there were side effects, they were manageable when monitored and treated. Some of the more serious side effects included fever, weight gain, shortness of breath, muscle pain in 23 percent of patients, and increased levels of white blood cells in half the patients. Gastrointestinal distress, fatigue, edema, cough, rash, headaches, and dizziness were also common side effects. They did not require interruption of therapy, however.

Trisenox is administered intravenously in two phases: induction therapy consisting of daily injections until the bone marrow is cleared of leukemic cells, for up to a maximum of 60 days. Then, consolidation therapy uses the same dose for 25 days beginning three weeks after bone marrow remission is evident.

Arsenic trioxide is also being studied for use in liver cancer, cervical cancer, multiple myeloma, and cancer of the prostate.

Treatments for Chronic Lymphocytic Leukemia

The 30,800 new cases of leukemia detected each year in the United States are almost equally divided between the acute and chronic forms of the disease. Leukemias are named by the rate of progression and the type of white blood cell involved. Acute leukemia progresses rapidly and can overwhelm your body in weeks or months.

Chronic lymphocytic leukemia (CLL) is the most common of the chronic leukemias and usually strikes in middle or old age and more men than women. Sometimes no treatment is necessary, but combination chemotherapy is the standard. Monoclonal antibodies are being investigated and one of them, Campath, has FDA approval for patients with CLL, who have been treated with alkylating agents and have failed therapy.

Intravenous immunoglobulin is given to prevent infection. Bone marrow transplantation may be indicated for younger patients.

MONOCLONAL ANTIBODIES FOR LYMPHOMA

Rituxan

In November 1997, Rituxan was approved for marketing by the FDA as a single agent for the treatment of relapsed or refractory low-grade or follicular, CD20-positive, B cell non-Hodgkin's lymphoma (NHL). Developed and co-promoted by Genentech, Inc. and IDEC Pharmaceuticals Corporation, Rituxan is the first new single-agent therapy in ten years for NHL and the first monoclonal antibody licensed for the treatment of cancer in the United States.

In May 1998 Genentech and IDEC announced the results of a small Phase II investigational pilot study combining Rituxan with standard chemotherapy. This pilot study revealed an overall response rate of 97 percent in patients with previously untreated intermediate- or high-grade NHL.

Rituxan is made from a genetically engineered mouse antibody designed to be a more specific treatment. Scientists don't know exactly how it works, but ultimately these antibodies zero in on the white blood cells involved in non-Hodgkin's lymphoma and trigger their death.

Rituxan has some risks, however. It can kill healthy white blood cells as well as cancerous ones, meaning patients could suffer infections although no unusual rates have appeared so far, according to Dr. Peter McLaughlin of the M. D. Anderson Cancer Center, the drug's lead investigator. Those cells grow back on their own within a year. Additionally, most patients have temporary and mild flulike symptoms, such as fever and chills, one to two hours after the first infusion, as their bodies learn to recognize the new antibody, he said.

Cells in the lymphatic system are programmed to do a specific job. When they become abnormal and are no longer able to do the job, they begin to divide and replicate themselves to form a tumor.

Lymphomas are cancers of the lymphatic system, a network of small vessels called lymphatics that return fluid from the tissues of the body to the bloodstream. The lymphatic system helps the body fight infection. Most of the cells in the lymphatic system are white blood cells, or lymphocytes. The abnormal cells congregate and enlarge the lymph nodes, which then form solid tumors in the body, or, on rare occasions, circulate in the blood. There are two primary categories of lymphoma: Hodgkin's disease and non-Hodgkin's lymphoma.

Hodgkin's disease is uncommon and has a cure rate of 95 percent. As the disease progresses, the body is less able to fight off infection, and flulike symptoms set in. Lymph nodes in the neck, armpit, and groin become enlarged and tumors develop. The cause of Hodgkin's disease is unknown, but it is suspected that a defect in the body's immune system couples with an outside stimulant—perhaps a virus. Hodgkin's disease usually responds well to treatment with radiation, chemotherapy, or both. Bone marrow transplantation plus high-dose chemotherapy with or without radiation is the treatment when the disease has relapsed.

Non-Hodgkin's lymphoma can show up anywhere in the body and often has primary sites outside the lymphatic system, such as the gastrointestinal tract. It can also involve the meninges (coverings of the brain) and the cerebrospinal fluid. The symptoms are similar to those of Hodgkin's disease. Chronic disorders of the immune system or the chronic use of drugs to suppress the immune system can predispose someone to lymphoma. People with AIDS are at higher risk. Aggressive lymphomas are increasingly seen in HIV-positive patients whose treatment requires special consideration.

About 240,000 Americans have non-Hodgkin's lymphoma. Many patients are successfully treated. But about half of them have an incurable form called low-grade NHL that causes repeated relapses over six or seven years. These patients try high doses of chemotherapy, radiation, and bone marrow transplants that can cause severe side effects, particularly when these treatments also kill healthy cells that get in the way.

Since the early 1970s, the incidence rates for NHL have nearly doubled, although the rate of increase began to slow during the 1990s. At the same time, the incidence of Hodgkin's disease has declined, particularly among the elderly. Before 1970, few people with Hodgkin's disease or non-Hodgkin's lymphoma survived. Now 50 to 80 percent survive. More people now die of complications of the treatment than of the disease.

Treatment of non-Hodgkin's lymphoma depends on the histologic type and stage. Many of the improvements in survival have been made using clinical trials that have attempted to improve on the best available accepted therapy. Even though standard treatment in patients with lymphomas can cure a significant fraction, numerous clinical trials that explore improvements in treatment are in progress. If possible, patients should be included in these studies.

Thousands of patients with an incurable type of non-Hodgkin's lymphoma now have their first new weapon against this disease in more than a decade. This genetically engineered drug attacks the immune system cancer with far fewer side effects than standard treatment. Rituxan is not a cure, but the FDA said it has an excellent success rate in shrinking tumors safely.

For patients today, Rituxan promises to buy some time. Rituxan therapy does not require hospitalization, but a complete course of four weekly transfusions will cost roughly $9,000, which is comparable to many chemotherapies. For full prescribing information on Rituxan, call 800-821-8590.

Rituxan Plus Zevalin

Lymphoma tumors are very sensitive to radiation, but targeting external beam radiation to cancerous immune system cells throughout the body is difficult. IDEC is developing a complementary product to Rituxan called Zevalin. This investigational therapy seeks to combine the targeting power of monoclonal antibodies with the cancer-killing ability of radiation. Zevalin is a murine monoclonal antibody that targets the CD20 antigen, like Rituxan. There's a difference, however. A connecting agent links this antibody to the radioisotope yttrium-90. In ongoing clinical studies, Zevalin is used in conjunction with Rituxan to treat patients with B cell NHL.

In December 2000, Thomas E. Witzig, M.D., of the Mayo Clinic reported on a Phase III controlled study of 143 patients with relapsed refractory low-grade non-Hodgkins' lymphoma. He noted that Zevalin combined with Rituxan showed an overall response rate of 80 percent compared to Rituxan alone, which showed an overall response rate of 56 percent. If approved by the FDA, Zevalin would be one of the first radioimmunotherapies available for commercial use in the United States.

LymphoCide

If Rituxan doesn't work for some people with NHL, there is another therapy in development at the biopharmaceutical company

Immunomedics. CEO Dr. Cindy Sullivan says, "Another therapy is needed for Rituxan failure. Any agents that are coming through will expand the lymphoma market. Combination therapy is well accepted, especially with antibodies."

The year 2000 proved to be a turnaround for treatment of NHL. This resulted from the encouraging results gained with Immunomedics' most advanced therapy, epratuzumab (LymphoCide), which is a humanized antibody directed against the CD22 marker of B cell lymphomas, including NHL. Approximately 30 percent of patients with the aggressive form of NHL (about 55 percent) can be cured by chemotherapy.

Unfortunately, the others with this aggressive form and all of those in the so-called indolent variety are not cured, so they get many courses of therapy. Epratuzumab appears to be tolerated well, has a convenient 30- to 60-minute infusion time, and shows very encouraging activity in several forms of NHL. There has been long-term complete response by people who did not respond to other aggressive therapies.

Immunomedics will continue clinical development in North America, and the company has licensed LymphoCide to Amgen.

Bexxar

Bexxar (iodine 131 tositumomab), produced by Corixa Corporation, is a radiolabeled monoclonal antibody being tested in clinical trials. Bexxar use is targeted for late-stage or low-grade B cell NHL patients. It is currently in Phase III clinical trials at multiple centers in the United States. FDA approval has been turned down until additional information is available.

Bexxar is an antibody with the radioactive iodine 131 attached. The drug attaches to a protein found only on the surface of B lymphocytes such as cancerous B cells found in many forms of NHL. The radioactivity targets the B cell and destroys it.

In Phase III trials, researchers found that all patients had more than a 50 percent shrinkage in their tumors. Bexxar is manufactured jointly by Corixa and GlaxoSmithKline Beecham.

Pretarget Technology

Pretarget technology, developed by NeoRx, may be able to deliver an unprecedented dose of radiation to lymphoma patients without the need for a costly stem cell transplant. Pretarget technology allows for various combinations of tumor-specific antibodies and therapeutic agents. Each combination can represent a potential new cancer therapy. By changing antibodies, different cancers may be treated. By changing therapeutic molecules, different cancer-killing agents may be delivered. The foundation for this new technology was created at Stanford University. NeoRx has the patent.

ANGIOGENESIS INHIBITORS FOR MULTIPLE MYELOMA

Multiple myeloma is a cancer that causes widespread bone destruction because the body makes too many antibodies. In 90 percent of multiple myeloma cases, cancerous plasma cells are found in the bone marrow. The cancer cells crowd out the red blood cells and cause anemia. This can also cause the bone to break down. Occasionally in the bone, plasma cells are concentrated in small tumors called plasmacytomas.

The growth of multiple myeloma is stimulated by interleukin-6 (IL-6), a hormone released by certain bone marrow cells. Treatments that block the action of this hormone are currently being investigated. Because IL-6 stimulates angiogenesis (blood vessel growth), thalidomide, a drug that may inhibit angiogenesis, may be beneficial.

Thalidomide

Thalidomide became famous in the 1960s for causing birth defects when given to pregnant women. However, the value of this drug in treating cancer is now the subject of much discussion.

Researchers at the Arkansas Cancer Research Center, the Mayo Clinic, and M. D. Anderson Cancer Center presented data on clinical trials of thalidomide as a single agent and in combination for the treatment of multiple myeloma.

The Celgene Corporation intended to apply for approval for the drug in 2001. Results of clinical trials of newly diagnosed myeloma patients treated with thalidomide in combination with other agents were to be available, according to Celgene president Sol J. Barer, Ph.D.

Neovastat

Aeterna Labs, of Quebec, got the go-ahead for a Phase II trial using Neovastat in mutiple myeloma in December 2000. This therapy inhibits angiogenesis by targeting the very mechanisms that are involved in the progression of multiple myeloma, said Dr. Sundar Jagannath, professor of medicine at St. Vincent's Comprehensive Cancer Center in New York, principal investigator in this country.

About 120 patients with progressive multiple myeloma, the second most prevalent blood cancer, will participate in 20 hospitals in this country and Canada. Final results were expected by the summer of 2002. They hope for accelerated approval.

RADIATION THERAPY FOR MULTIPLE MYELOMA

Skeletal Targeted Radiotherapy

A Phase III trial began in October 2000 with skeletal targeted radiotherapy (STR) for the treatment of multiple myeloma. The principal investigators are Kenneth Anderson, M.D., of the Dana-Farber Cancer Institute in Boston and chairman of the Advisory Board of the Multiple Myeloma Research Foundation, and Richard Champlin, M.D., chief of the bone marrow transplant section at M. D. Anderson Cancer Center in Houston, Texas.

In Phase I and II trials, STR delivered high radiation doses to bone and bone marrow where multiple myeloma arises, without making the accompanying high-dose chemotherapy any more toxic. Previously, radiation treatment to the entire skeleton was limited to low doses of radiation. The breakthrough of STR is that it delivers high-dose radiation—about 4,000 rads—directly to the tumor and bone with minimal harm to other organs.

NeoRx, the Seattle company that developed the therapy, is conducting a Phase I and II trial in patients with multiple myeloma. In this trial, at the lowest doses, 12 of 27 patients achieved complete remission. In addition, because STR is well tolerated, the investigators decided to raise the age limit in future trials. A pivotal trial was initiated in 2000 at major cancer centers in North America.

"Previously reported safety and efficacy trends appear to be continuing," said Paul Abrams, M.D., J.D., NeoRx's CEO. "Results on patients not yet completed cannot be predicted. We are moving forward to initiate the Phase III trial that will randomize patients to standard therapy with STR versus standard therapy alone. This is an exciting time for patients and for the company."

Patients with multiple myeloma typically have a single protein present in their blood that represents the antibody made by the myeloma cells. The presence or absence of this protein can be measured by sophisticated biochemical techniques, and it must be undetectable for a patient to be deemed in a complete remission.

The American Cancer Society estimates 13,700 new cases and 11,400 deaths from multiple myeloma in the United States every year. Many patients with the disease are elderly and cannot be treated aggressively.

Holmium-166 DOTMP

NeoRx is also developing a novel radiopharmaceutical called holmium-166 DOTMP. It emits high-energy beta particles that can destroy cells. DOTMP binds to bone and carries holmium to the bone and adjacent bone marrow. Because radiation is selectively delivered to the site of the disease, the exposure to normal organs is reduced compared to conventional external beam body irradiation. This agent is designed to treat cancers that arise in the bone or bone marrow, as well as those that spread to the bone and bone marrow, such as breast and prostate cancers.

CONVENTIONAL TREATMENTS FOR MULTIPLE MYELOMA

The cause of multiple myeloma is unknown, but it generally occurs in people over 50. The average age at diagnosis is 70. It is about twice as common among African Americans as white Americans. The disease can be treated but not cured.

Although surgery may be used in certain cases, the most common treatment for multiple myeloma is chemotherapy, usually with a combination of drugs. Patients also are treated with bisphosphonates, which cause the bone to be resistant to damage from myeloma. The standard bisphosphonate used to treat multiple myeloma patients is pamidronate, which is given intravenously. Another bisphosphonate, clodronate, can be given in pills, but often causes upset stomach. Newer bisphosphonates, zoledronate and ibandronate, are currently being evaluated.

Interferon actually slows the growth of multiple myeloma. It seems to work best in patients that have had chemotherapy and are in remission. Interferon seems to prolong the remission but has serious side effects.

Autologous bone marrow transplantation, using the patient's own bone marrow, is being studied in clinical trials, as is peripheral blood stem cell transplant. The patient's blood is passed through a machine that removes the stem cells (immature blood cells) and returned to the patient. Meanwhile, the stem cells are then treated with drugs to kill the cancer cells and frozen until they are put back in the patient.

Plasmapheresis is a treatment that removes blood from a patient's vein and separates the blood cells from the blood plasma, although it doesn't kill the cancer cells. Rather, it relieves some of the symptoms of the disease. The blood cells are later returned into another vein and the plasma, which contains the abnormal antibody protein produced by the myeloma cells, is replaced with a salt solution and blood proteins from donors.

WHERE TO FIND INFORMATION ABOUT LEUKEMIA, LYMPHOMA, AND MULTIPLE MYELOMA

Cure for Lymphoma Foundation
215 Lexington Avenue
New York, NY 10016
Hotline: 800-CFL-6848
Telephone: 212-213-9595
Fax: 212-213-1987
Web site: www.clf.org
E-mail: infoclf@clf.org
This organization provides education and advocacy, and supports research.

International Myeloma Foundation
12650 Riverside Drive
North Hollywood, CA 91607
Hotline: 800-452-CURE
Telephone: 800-452-2873
Fax: 818-487-7454
Web site: www.myeloma.org
Provides information, support, as well as information on clinical trials.

The Leukemia & Lymphoma Society
1311 Mamaroneck Avenue
White Plains, NY 10605
Telephone: 914-949-5213
Information Resource Center: 800-955-4572
Web site: www.leukemia-lymphoma.org
A source of educational information about leukemia, lymphoma,

Hodgkin's lymphoma, and myeloma. In addition, this group provides programs, support, and booklets.

Lymphoma Research Foundation of America
8800 Venice Boulevard
Los Angeles, CA 90034
Telephone: 310-204-7040
Fax: 310-204-7043
Web site: www.lymphoma.org
   This organization provides education and advocacy, and supports research.

ONGOING CLINICAL TRIALS FOR LEUKEMIA, LYMPHOMA, AND MULTIPLE MYELOMA

There are literally hundreds of clinical trials in various stages of development around the world. To list them all here would be misleading because by the time you read this book, some trials may have closed and many others may have opened. Clinical trials have specific eligibility requirements that may eliminate many cancer patients. The few trials listed here are only a sampling of the trials that may be open to you. The best way to locate clinical trials appropriate for your situation is to ask your doctor, check the web sites listed in Chapter 4, and call the biotech companies listed in Appendix C.

Ongoing Clinical Trials for Leukemia

1. A Phase I study of the recombinant immunotoxin LMB-2 in patients with TAC-expressing leukemias and lymphomas. Contact Robert Kreitman, Division of Basic Sciences, Laboratory of Molecular Biology, Bethesda, MD, at 301-496-6947.
2. A Phase I study of CD40-activated autologous tumor cell vaccine in patients with B cell acute lymphoblastic leukemia

(ALL). This will determine the feasibility of generating a vaccine comprising this vaccine. It's a multicenter study. The ALL cells are harvested, cultured with CD40 ligand, pulsed with keyhole limpet hemocyanin, and then irradiated.

Contact W. Nicholas Haining at the Dana-Farber Cancer Institute in Boston at 617-632-5923.

3. A Phase I study of monoclonal antibody Hu1D10 in patients with previously treated chronic lymphocytic leukemia, small lymphocytic lymphoma, or acute lymphoblastic leukemia. Dose escalation will determine the maximum tolerated dose or effective dose of this therapy. It's a multicenter study.

Contact Pierluigi Porcu of the Arthur James Cancer Hospital at Ohio State University at 614-293-4275.

4. A Phase I trial of yttrium Y90 humanized monoclonal antibody M195 and etoposide followed by stem cell transplantation in patients with refractory leukemias. It will determine the maximum tolerated dose of the therapy.

Contact Peter Maslak at Memorial Sloan-Kettering Cancer Center in New York at 212-639-5518.

5. A Phase II study of arsenic trioxide in patients with recurrent or refractory acute lymphoblastic leukemia or refractory blastic phase chronic myelogenoous leukemia. The study will determine the response in patients with Philadelphia chromosone-positive recurrent or refractory ALL.

Contact Kapil Narain Bhalla at the H. Lee Moffitt Cancer Center and Research Institute in Tampa, FL, at 813-903-6861.

Ongoing Clinical Trials for Lymphoma

1. A Phase I trial of the monoclonal antibody HuM291 in patients with advanced or recurrent T cell lymphomas. This is a dose escalation study, which means that patients with a partial or complete response to the therapy will receive escalating doses until the maximum is reached.

This is an NCI trial with Stanford University Medical Center. Contact Youn Kim at 650-723-7893 at Stanford.

Ongoing Clinical Trials for Multiple Myeloma

1. A Phase I/II study of arsenic trioxide plus ascorbic acid in patients with recurrent or refractory multiple myeloma. The purpose is to determine the maximum tolerated dose of arsenic trioxide when its is administered with ascorbic acid. It is a multicenter study. Patients receive arsenic trioxide intravenously over one to four hours and ascorbic acid intravenously over five to ten minutes on days 1 to 5 weekly for five weeks. Treatment continues every seven weeks for up to six courses in the absence of disease progression or unacceptable toxicity. A total of 31 to 43 patients will be accrued for this study over two and a half years.

    Contact Kelvin Lee at Sylvester Cancer Center at the University of Miami at 305-243-1044. Several other locations in Miami are involved in the study.

2. A Phase II randomized study of bevacizumab with or without thalidomide in patients with relapsed or refractory multiple myeloma. This is a multicenter study that was approved as of this writing, but not yet active.

    Contact George Somlo at Beckman Research Institute, City of Hope, Duarte, California, at 626-359-8111.

3. A Phase II trial of AE-941 (Neovastat: shark cartilage) in patients with early relapse or refractory multiple myeloma. This study will determine the confirmed tumor response rate and safety of patients with this disease treated with Neovastat. This is a multicenter study and patients will take the drug orally twice a day. Up to 125 patients will be enrolled.

    Contact Pierre Champagne at Aeterna Laboratories in Quebec, Canada, at 888-349-3232.

4. A Phase II study of arsenic trioxide in a total of 55 patients with multiple myeloma.

    Contact Carolyn Paradise at Cell Therapeutics at 206-270-8441. Other contacts include James Ronald Mason at Scripps Clinic in La Jolla, CA, at 858-554-8597; Robert Rivkin of the Rocky Mountain Cancer Center in Denver at 303-285-5087;

Farhad Ravandi of the University of Illinois at Chicago at 312-996-5982; Mohamad Ahmed Hussein of the Cleveland Clinic Taussig Cancer Center at 216-445-6830; Gary E. Goodman of the Swedish Cancer Institute in Seattle at 206-386-2122.

CHAPTER 12

▼

BREAKTHROUGH TREATMENTS FOR MELANOMA

The best first step in treating melanoma is to gather as much information about this disease as possible. A substantial amount of melanoma-related research is in progress, and there have been significant advancements in understanding and treating patients with melanoma.

Melanoma, the deadliest form of skin cancer, has been on the rise for decades, perhaps because of damage to the ozone layer in the atmosphere. It is increasing at about 4 percent a year, faster than any other type of cancer, and is now the seventh most common cancer in the United States. If the alarming rates of skin cancer continue, nearly half of all Americans who live to 65 will develop some form of skin cancer. It is the most frequent cancer occurring in women between 25 and 29 years of age. After breast cancer, it is the second most frequent cancer in women from 30 to 34. By the end of the 20th century, the chance of getting skin cancer over a lifetime in this country was 1 in 75.

Every year in the United States, approximately 1,300,000 new cases of the highly curable squamous and basal cell cancers are reported. Most often, they are found among light-skinned people.

Melanoma, which accounts for about 4 percent of cancer cases,

178

accounts for 79 percent of the deaths. In 2000, nearly 48,000 Americans—130 a day—were diagnosed with melanoma. In the year 2001, there were an estimated 10,000 deaths from the disease in the United States, and 770 in Canada. Men are two or three times as likely to get skin cancer as women, and whites are ten times more vulnerable than African Americans.

The National Cancer Institute estimates that at any one time about half a million Americans have melanoma. If detected when it is still limited to one site on the skin, melanoma can usually be cured with surgery. Once it has spread beyond the local site into the lymph system, it is considered Stage III disease. When the melanoma has spread to other parts of the body, it is Stage IV.

Because most skin cancers can be cured in their early stages, an early diagnosis is critical. Symptoms of skin cancer may include any change in the appearance or sensation of the skin—for example, a change in the size or color of a mole or other dark growth or spot. Itchiness, tenderness, and pain are also symptoms.

Skin conditions that need to be watched are actinic keratosis and Bowen's disease, because both can become cancer. Actinic keratosis is a thickening of the skin. Most often, this is found in older people with longtime exposure to the sun. Bowen's disease can appear on parts of the body not exposed to the sun. It may be caused by a wart virus.

Other than sun exposure and having fair skin, risk factors for skin cancer may include occupational exposure to coal tar, pitch, creosote, arsenic compounds, or radium. A family history of the disease and having multiple moles can also put you at risk.

Basal cell carcinomas, the most common skin cancer, grow slowly and rarely spread internally. Such carcinomas are ulcerated areas on the face, neck, and upper back. They have a rolled edge and a pearly appearance. If they are not treated they can ulcerate and bleed. While they can invade the bone and cartilage, they rarely metastasize.

Squamous cell carcinoma is less common than basal, but occasionally spreads to the lymph nodes. It is red, scaly, sharply outlined, and appears on the face, ears, neck, forearms, and backs of the hand. It's caused by chronic sun or high doses of X-rays or poorly healed wounds. This one can metastasize if it is left untreated.

Of the five main treatment options for these two types of skin cancer, surgery is most often the treatment of choice. Destroying the lesion with radiation, laser, heat, or cold are also options. Some advanced cases may also require chemotherapy.

Kaposi's sarcoma is a type of skin cancer that used to be very rare, occurring only in people over 70 of Russian-Jewish, Italian, or African ancestry. But there has been a substantial increase associated with AIDS. It affects about a quarter of all AIDS patients.

Melanoma begins in melanocytes, the specialized skin cells that provide pigment to the skin. Melanomas often appear on the backs of men and on the legs of women. They usually start in the melanocytes or an existing mole. Melanomas are usually secondary to sun damage, but can appear in unexposed sites such as the mucous lining of the mouth, vagina, or anus. They appear as asymmetrical spots with a variation in color and ragged edges. When a mole changes, it can be the result of a melanoma. Blondes and redheads and people with freckles are the most vulnerable to melanoma. Intense sun exposure in childhood increases the risk.

TREATING MELANOMA

As with many cancers, early detection of melanoma is critical. When the disease is localized, most melanomas can be cured. It is essential to remove the primary growth completely. That may require the removal of nearby lymph nodes, too. Removal of all suspicious moles is critical.

Radiation therapy is generally used on skin cancers that cannot be surgically removed or when surgery would be too risky for the patient. Oral or intravenous chemotherapy is used with recurrent cancers or those that cannot be controlled with surgery or radiation.

However, the news is good with advanced melanoma because the cure rates keep rising as new discoveries yield varied and improved treatments. Surgery is much more effective than it used to be, and much less tissue is removed with the lesion. Ten years ago, if you had a melanoma on the back of your leg, a good chunk of your leg was cut out with the tumor.

Studies have shown that combining a number of chemotherapy drugs with one or more immunotherapy drugs (usually interferon alpha or interleukin-2) is more effective than a single drug. Drugs used to treat melanoma include dacarbazine (DTIC), carmustine (BCNU), and cisplatin. The combination of these three drugs with tamoxifen is called the Dartmouth Regimen. Another combination for treating melanoma is cisplatin, vincristine, and dacarbazine.

IMMUNOTHERAPY

No proven life-prolonging therapy exists for metastatic malignant melanoma. The response rate with the current drug of choice, DTIC, is about 20 percent and usually of short duration. However, combining a number of chemotherapy drugs with one or more immunotherapy drugs (usually interferon alpha or interleukin-2) is more effective than a single drug.

The FDA approved the combination of Proleukin and dacarbazine as a first choice in treating appropriate patients with metastatic melanoma. Studies showed good response rates from total reduction of all tumors to improved survival.

Dacarbazine is typically given intravenously once a day for up to ten days and repeated every three or four weeks. Tumors shrink and extend survival time.

Proleukin

The FDA has approved use of high-dose IL-2 (Proleukin) for Stage IV melanoma. This immunological therapy makes use of naturally occurring chemicals in your body. Proleukin boosts the production and activity of several important immune system cells. These include T cells (T4 and T8), B cells that produce antibodies, macrophages, and natural killer cells (NK cells).

Proleukin is the first drug approved by the FDA in over 20 years for the treatment of metastatic melanoma. (It is also the only therapy approved for patients with metastatic renal cell carcinoma.) Proleukin offers the possibility of long-lasting remission. High-dose IL-2 has an overall response rate of about 16 percent.

In clinical trials of Proleukin, 16 percent of patients responded to the drug and approximately half of them remain alive over four years after treatment. Proleukin produced a complete response in 6 percent of patients. This means the tumors disappeared. About 60 percent of the patients who had this complete response have remained in remission for more than five years without further treatment. While not all patients did that well, the study shows that the drug obviously works in many patients.

For more information about Proleukin, call Chiron's Professional Services Group at 800-CHIRON-8 (800-244-7668).

Intron A

Schering-Plough's recombinant interferon alpha, Intron A, is another interferon molecule used extensively in the treatment of cancer. It is currently approved in the United States for four cancers including melanoma. Intron A was approved in 1995 in the United States and two years later in Europe.

The results of a clinical trial, reported in Europe in 2000, confirm the use of Intron A for adjuvant treatment of adults with high-risk malignant melanoma. The study reaffirms the consistent effectiveness of Intron A, according to John M. Kirkwood, M.D., director of the Melanoma Center at the University of Pittsburgh Cancer Institute. Intron A is the only adjuvant therapy that has prolonged life for people at high risk of relapse.

Melanoma Vaccines

Antimelanoma vaccine therapy is being tested. One of the most promising new treatments involves the addition of certain genes to the cancer cells. This can be done in one of three ways:

- Using a virus to inject a specific gene into melanoma cells and making the melanoma sensitive to a drug that usually does not affect the cancer
- Replacing some of the damaged genes in the melanoma that cause the cells to grow and metastasize
- Adding certain genes to melanoma cells, which are then used for vaccine therapy

One basic idea behind anticancer vaccines is to isolate an antigen—that is, a unique feature on the surface of the cancer cell—and then to mass-produce this antigen and inject it back into the cancer patient. In theory, once the immune system "recognizes" the antigen, it should trigger the policing mechanisms to target the tumor for destruction.

Anticancer vaccines are still a largely unproven technology, and the various companies in this niche face years of safety and efficacy experiments. But there is reason for hope. Avax Technologies of Kansas City, Missouri, recently began selling an anticancer vaccine for melanoma in Australia and is close to selling the same product in Germany and the Netherlands. Avax CEO Jeffrey Jonas said it may be three or four years before his company completes the experiments needed to win approval in the United States.

Avax makes vaccine from the patient's own tumor cells, collected after surgical removal of the tumor. Doctors who wish to treat their patients with melanoma vaccine (MVAX) send removed tumors to the company's facility in Sydney, Australia, for storage. At the time of treatment, tumor cells are used to create an individualized cancer vaccine. It is then administered systemically on an outpatient basis once a week for seven weeks. Six months later, the patient gets a booster shot.

MVAX was administered to 37 people with Stage IV melanoma. They had undergone complete resection of tumors that had spread to various internal organs. The two-year survival was 60 percent, with an overall rate of 27 months or more, nearly double that of the best comparable data that show a 15-month survival with surgery alone. The safety profile of MVAX in these patients, for whom there is no standard therapy, is excellent, with only a local response at vaccine infection sites. More than 400 patients have received the vaccine.

David Berd, M.D., professor of medicine at Thomas Jefferson University in Philadelphia, led the study. He said that in 25 of the 37 people, cancer had spread to vital organs, mainly the lung. Since the tumor had already spread through the body, MVAX was administered after complete surgery resection of the metastasized organ. A single injection is given followed by a single low dose of cyclophosphamide, followed by six weekly injections of vaccine mixed with BCG, a helper for the immune system.

Fusion Cell Technology

Genzyme Molecular Oncology, a Cambridge, Massachusetts, biotech company, has been working with Dr. Steven Rosenberg at the National Cancer Institute to come up with a way to treat this disease. The company has developed a melanoma tumor vaccine that uses the body's own white cells to fight the tumor. Fifty-four patients with late-stage metastatic disease were treated with this vaccine. And 32 percent have shown objective cancer responses.

Genzyme initiated Phase I and II clinical trials in melanoma in October 2000. Lead investigators are Donald Kufe, M.D., professor of medicine at the Dana-Farber Cancer Institute and Harvard Medical School; David Avigan, M.D., director of the bone marrow transplant program at Beth Israel Deaconess Medical Center and Harvard Medical School; and Jianlin Gong, M.D., instructor of medicine at Dana-Farber and Harvard.

The trials will utilize a novel technology called dendritic/cancer cell fusion, developed by the three doctors. Genzyme has exclusively licensed this technology from Dana-Farber and is funding both trials.

The dendritic/cancer cell fusion technology combines a patient's dendritic cells—powerful immune stimulators—with their inactivated tumor cells in a chemical fusion procedure. The fused cells are injected back into the patient in order to stimulate an immune response against the patient's cancer.

About 20 patients with advanced metastatic melanoma were to be enrolled and treated in the study in Boston at Beth Israel Deaconess. People with advanced-stage melanoma who are interested in participating in the trials should contact Carolyn Stone in Dr. Avigan's office, 617-667-3029, for information.

Cell fusion technology eliminates the need to identify specific antigens for these vaccines because it incorporates the entire menu of antigens found on the original tumor to provide targets to the immune system, according to Dr. Kufe.

Genzyme also initiated Phase I and II clinical trials of a gene therapy cancer vaccine for melanoma. This in vivo vaccine combines two of the most widely expressed melanoma tumor antigens, MelanA/MART-I and gp100. The vaccine will employ an adenovirus vector to deliver the antigens between the layers of the skin.

Frank G. Haluska, M.D., Ph.D., at the Massachusetts General Hospital Cancer Center, is the lead investigator of the trial to be conducted at his hospital and U.S. Oncology in Dallas. Approximately 36 patients with Stage II, III, or IV melanoma who have already had surgery are in the study.

The ex vivo trial takes cells from the patient's immune system and ensures that those cells contain the vaccine before reintroducing them into the patient's body. The new in vivo trial will take the next step toward commercialization by delivering the vaccine directly to the patient. It will rely on Genzyme gene delivery technology to deliver the vaccine to the appropriate cells in the immune system.

"We have designed the in vivo melanoma trial to help skin cancer patients mount a strong immune system response to their tumor, and to enable us to obtain gene delivery data that will help us develop cancer vaccines for a range of cancers," said Mark Goldberg, M.D.

According to Dr. Haluska, the observations of immune response in molecular targeted therapy, though preliminary, are very encouraging. He said that by engaging the immune system's innate ability to find and destroy cancer cells, a successful gene therapy cancer vaccine for melanoma would offer patients a less invasive alternative to current treatments like chemotherapy, with few if any side effects.

If you have these stages of melanoma, call for information for the trial at 617-724-7081 in Boston or 214-370-1822 in Dallas.

ANTISENSE THERAPY

Patients with advanced melanoma also respond to a new antisense drug, according to a study presented at the American Association for Cancer Research meeting in April 2000. During the Phase I toxicity and dosing trial, doctors observed a complete remission of melanoma in a 90-year-old woman with Stage IV disease.

"To our knowledge, this is the first demonstration of clinical response, including complete disappearance of disease, using an antisense therapy for solid tumors," said Burkhard Jansen, M.D., associate professor of clinical pharmacology at the University of Vienna. The trial is also the first to demonstrate that an antisense drug can successfully attack its target in patients' cancer cells at the molecular level.

Double-stranded DNA is composed of one sense strand and one antisense strand. Together they function as a system of checks and balances in the multistep process that unleashes disease. A code embedded in the sense strand leads to production of a particular RNA and protein. The complementary antisense strand can prevent expression of the gene encoded by its strand-mate, leaving the genetic information intact but unable to operate.

In the Austrian study, scientists used an antisense drug called G3139, provided by Genta, to turn off BCL2 gene function. Expression of BCL2 is associated with resistance to chemotherapy, suggesting that it may act as a shield to repel anticancer drugs or blunt their impact.

According to the researchers, patients with advanced melanoma received both G3139 and the antimelanoma drug dacarbazine. Most of the patients had failed to respond to other treatments, including dacarbazine. The combination regimen produced responses in 6 of 14 patients—43 percent—some lasting more than a year. Of the responses, one was complete, two were partial, and three were minor. Two other patients had evidence of antitumor activity with stabilized disease. Antitumor activity was even seen in some patients after failure of other dacarbazine treatment programs. Tests showed that as BCL2 protein levels dropped in the tumor cells, more melanoma cells died. Side effects, including fever, rash, and short-term changes in liver function in some patients, were tolerated and did not require changes in the administered doses of chemotherapy.

By breaching one suspected defense of malignant cells, G3139 appears to have allowed a standard cancer therapy to work much more effectively. A Phase III trial has been organized in Europe and North America by Genta to evaluate this novel approach in a larger patient population.

EXPERIMENTAL TREATMENTS

Zadaxin Plus Chemotherapy

A SciClone Pharmaceuticals study published in the journal *Melanoma Research* suggests that Zadaxin (thymalfasin), SciClone's lead immunotherapy, increases the effectiveness of chemotherapy for metastatic malignant melanoma.

In the Phase II study of 20 people with Stage IV and V melanoma, there was a response rate of 50 percent to the combination of Zadaxin, dacarbazine (DTIC), and interferon. Five patients had a complete response and five a partial response. Five patients survived for more than two years and two patients survived for more than five years. No additional side effects were observed by adding Zadaxin to their treatment.

DTIC therapy significantly depresses the patient's immune system. In the study, Zadaxin significantly improved the immune system by restoring their natural killer cells and helper T cells, both of which are disease-fighting white blood cells.

Donald R. Sellers, SciClone's president and CEO, reported that he believes Zadaxin immunotherapy will be a key component of multiple drug treatments for numerous cancers.

Zadaxin enhances the immune system's ability to recognize and destroy cancerous cells. It is a key component in the growing trend toward multiple drug cocktails for cancer and infectious diseases. Zadaxin is in late-stage development for cancer worldwide. It is now approved for marketing in 19 countries, mostly for the treatment of hepatitis C.

Allovectin 7

Vical, a company in San Diego, develops drugs based on patented DNA gene transfer technologies for the prevention and treatment of life-threatening diseases. Current focus is on immune response against cancer. They have retained all rights to their lead immunotherapy drug, Allovectin 7. It is in Phase II and Phase III trials for patients with advanced melanoma.

Allovectin 7 is designed to stimulate the patient's immune system to attack the melanoma. It works by replacing a key protein (MHC class I protein) that is often missing or not adequately present on the surface of most cancer cells. The absence of this key protein makes many melanomas "invisible" to the immune system. After treatment with Allovectin 7, this key protein is replaced with a similar protein known as HLA-B7. As a result, the patient's immune system is now able to recognize and attack the melanoma. Interestingly, Allovectin 7 can achieve this with very little in the way of side effects.

Previous clinical trials showed the drug to reduce tumors in some patients. Tumor shrinkage was noted more often in patients with soft tissue disease, like skin and lymph nodes, than in those with internal organs affected, like the liver and lung.

Isolated Limb Perfusion

Isolated limb perfusion is an experimental chemotherapy used to treat melanomas on arms or legs. It involves temporarily separating the circulation of the affected limb from the body and injecting high doses of chemotherapy into the artery feeding the limb. This therapy, along with the use of cytokines or granulocyte stimulating factors (GMF-CSF) have been incompletely studied in the adjuvant setting for melanoma. There are current trials ongoing that are investigating the potential of GMF-CSF or cytokines like interferon, which regulate the immune system. Eastern Cooperative Oncology Group and the Southwestern Cooperative Oncology Group are conducting trials.

WHERE TO FIND INFORMATION ABOUT MELANOMA

The Skin Cancer Foundation
P.O. Box 561
New York, NY 10156
212-725-5176
Telephone: 800-SKIN-490 (754-6490)
Web site: www.skincancer.org
E-mail: info@skincancer.org
   This group provides education and awareness to the public. They may be able to help you find resources in your own community.

ONGOING CLINICAL TRIALS FOR MELANOMA

   There are literally hundreds of clinical trials in various stages of development around the world. To list them all here would be misleading because by the time you read this book, some trials may have closed and many others may have opened. Clinical trials have specific eligibility requirements that may eliminate many cancer patients. The few trials listed here are only a sampling of the trials that may be open to you. The best way to locate clinical trials appropriate for your situation is to ask your doctor, check the web sites listed in Chapter 4, and call the biotech companies listed in Appendix C.

1. A Phase I trial to compare the effectiveness of melanoma vaccine with or without sargramostim in treating patients who have Stage IV malignant melanoma. Two groups of patients will be treated with injections of the vaccine, but one group will also get the sargramostim. The vaccine is comprised of tyrosinase peptide, gp100 antigen, and MART-1:27-35 antigen emulsified in montanide ISA-51.

   Contact: This is an NCI trial at the Mayo Clinic in Rochester, MN. Call Svetomir Markovic at 507-284-3903.

2. A Phase I trial to study the effectiveness of vaccine therapy in treating patients who have metastasized cancer that has not responded to previous therapy. Two groups of patients will receive injections of vaccine, but one group will also receive interleukin-2. The vaccine is MAGE-12 peptide.

   Contact: This is an NCI study chaired by Francesco M. Marincola of the Center for Cancer Research in Bethesda, MD, at 301-496-0997.

3. A Phase I trial to study the effectiveness of vaccine therapy in treating patients with Stage IV melanoma. White blood cells will be collected and patients will then be assigned to one of three groups. One group will receive three infusions of vaccine. In the second group patients will receive three or six injections of vaccine. Those in group three will receive the injection into the lymph nodes.

   Contact: NCI and the University of Pennsylvania Cancer Center. Contact Brian J. Czerniecki at 215-662-4392 in Philadelphia.

4. A Phase I trial to study the effectiveness of vaccine therapy in treating patients with metastasized melanoma. Vaccine will be made from the patient's white blood cells. Patients will receive injections of filgrastim once a day for six days. Then blood cells will be collected and teated in the lab to make the vaccine. Patients will receive an injection of the vaccine once every two weeks for eight weeks, then in gradually decreasing time frames.

   This is an NCI and Baylor University Medical Center trial.

Contact Joseph Wayne Fay at 214-820-2610 at Baylor in Dallas.

5. A Phase I trial to study the effectiveness of biological therapy combined with temozolomide in treating patients with metastasized melanoma. Patients' white blood cells will be collected and treated in the lab with monoclonal antibodies, interleukin-2, and interleukin-12. Eventually, patients will also receive temozolomide and an infusion of the treated white blood cells.

   This is an NCI trial with St. Luke's Medical Center in Milwaukee, WI. Contact John P. Hanson Jr. at 414-385-3086.

6. A Phase I/II trial to study the effectiveness of temozolomide plus thalidomide in treating patients who have Stage III or IV melanoma that cannot be removed during surgery.

   This is an NCI trial with Memorial Sloan-Kettering Cancer Center in New York. Contact Paul B. Chapman at 212-639-5015.

CHAPTER 13

▼

A LIFETIME OF VIGILANCE
High-Tech Diagnostic Testing

Each year in this country an estimated 1.2 million people are diagnosed with cancer. More than half a million died of it in 2001. The disease, which costs the economy $107 billion a year, according to the National Institutes of Health, is often curable if it is detected at an early stage, when it is organ-confined and there are no or few symptoms.

Even when cancer is cured once, there is always the chance that it will return—that your cells once again may decide to run amok. For this reason, it is essential to regularly monitor for any hint of cancer for the rest of your life. Also, you may be cured of one cancer, only to develop some other cancer later. As you age and your cells break down, you are vulnerable. Having one cancer also puts you at higher risk for others. In addition to regular checkups with your doctor, and staying aware of changes in your body, there are many diagnostic procedures you should be aware of.

Technology has made it possible for us to characterize the structure and function of genes and the cellular process. We can check blood for signs of cancer cells. We can literally photograph and examine everything inside the body. For example, endoscopic testing puts a fiber-optic tube and camera inside your digestive canal and takes pictures. You can even watch it on a video monitor during the process.

What are the new tests and what do they discover? In addition to new blood tests for cancer such as the prostate-specific antigen (PSA) for prostate cancer, the emerging field of genetic tests for underlying and undetected cancers is beginning to have clinical significance. There's a number of diagnostic tests cancer patients should undergo, such as blood testing for tumor markers, radiology, and endoscopy.

Keep in mind, however, that existing tests lack specificity and accuracy and many are expensive and invasive, requiring physicians to slice or scrape tissue from patients. Nevertheless, there are more and better diagnostic tests that can be used to detect and monitor cancer.

THE NEW FRONTIER IN CANCER DETECTION

Medical researchers are predicting that soon they will have the tools to look inside tumors and collect their molecular characteristics the way a detective gathers fingerprints at the scene of a crime. Armed with a computer printout of abnormal cells, doctors would know whether the tumor would grow quickly or slowly, and whether it would spread to other parts of the body. And best of all, they would be able to know which treatments would chemically kill the tumor cells. This will grow even clearer as powerful new technologies give us the ability to explore in even greater detail the molecular characteristics of cancer.

Most people are surprised by the diagnosis of cancer. It's unexpected even though the cellular changes that lead to it have been developing slowly for decades. This discovery creates a window of opportunity to catch the cancer cells before they ever become a threat to your health. This could give us a way to prevent it from metastasizing.

We are working to identify early telltale changes in gene expres-

sion that indicate a developing tumor. This should lead us to identify many potential biomarkers from precancerous tumors throughout the body that, when grouped together, tell us more than an
individual biomarker.

Today, as an indication of the enormous technological strides
that science has taken in the last decade, large laboratories that
specialize in sequencing DNA can catalog a million bases of DNA
in a single day. Many of these technologies become standard tools
to see the molecular characterization of tumors. Some of these include:

- Chip technology. Computer chips arrayed with the full sequence of a known cancer gene will allow doctors to quickly
  test for gene mutations.
- DNA arrays. DNA arrays record the expression of hundreds
  of genes at once.
- Laser capture microdissection. This fully automated device
  lifts small clusters of tumor cells directly from a biopsy, for
  rapid analysis of gene expression of tumor cells.

Until now, it was always a trial-and-error method. However, as we
learn more about the molecular nature of tumor cells, we are also
beginning to explain the molecular causes of drug resistance. For
example, the lack of estrogen receptors on the surface of breast
tumor cells indicates that the tumor is not likely to respond to hormone therapy. New examples of molecular profiling are now ap-
pearing in the medical literature. They should in the coming years
help make diagnosis a more exact science. At the same time, molecular profiling will have great value in helping us know how to best
treat a patient.

WHAT TO KNOW ABOUT TUMOR MARKERS

One thing is important to remember when it comes to diagnostic tests for cancer. Only PSA, the prostate-specific antigen test for
cancer, is approved for diagnostic screening to find undiagnosed

cancer. And even in this case, a digital rectal exam is mandatory in confirming the diagnosis of prostate cancer. All other diagnostic tests for cancer, called tumor markers, are used to monitor the progress of the disease after diagnosis and the response to therapy. These are simple blood tests, but the lab must be alerted on what to look for.

The National Cancer Institute's (NCI) Cancer Genome Anatomy Project (CGAP) has enabled the discovery of literally hundreds of potential markers for cancer since the end of the 1990s. For example, in 1998 NCI knew of no potential unique markers for ovarian cancer, but by 1999, had provided 400 candidates ready to be tested.

The FDA has recently considered faster approval of tumor markers for use in the United States. Now there are only 6 markers approved here, but in Europe there are over 30 markers routinely used to help cancer patients. Always ask your doctor if there are any new tumor markers approved that may help you monitor your cancer.

Recently the marker CA27-29 was approved by the FDA for monitoring the recurrence of Stage II and III breast cancer. Markers can also identify the HER2/neu gene, estrogen and prostate hormone receptors, squamous cell antigen in skin cancer, and the p53 oncogene.

ON THE BIOTECH HORIZON

The Matritech NMP22 is a brand-new urine test to detect the recurrence of bladder cancer. The test identifies a protein that is released into the urine. The test is noninvasive, and it can aid in the diagnosis of people with symptoms or risk factors for transitional cell carcinoma (TCC) of the bladder in conjunction with standard diagnostic procedures. It can aid in identifying patients at risk for occult or rapidly recurring disease. The Matritech NMP22 Assay enables urologists to accurately predict residual or recurrent bladder cancer as soon as five days after surgical removal of a bladder tumor.

Many biotech companies have changed their focus toward developing more accurate and earlier biomarkers for cancer, rather than just improving automation and sensitivity on existing tests. That had been the tendency among diagnostics companies. These companies include the new Minerva Pharmaceuticals as well as newly created divisions of existing companies such as Millennium Predictive Medicine (MPMx), a division of Millennium Pharmaceuticals. These new hunters of diagnostic biomarkers hope to play a role beyond improving cancer diagnosis. They envision biomarkers that will allow more accurate disease-stage monitoring and characterization, more effective choice of therapy, and, ultimately, the development of therapies themselves.

Despite the plethora of new technologies, tools, and genomic data, however, cancer-specific markers have proven to be difficult beasts to catch, let alone to validate and turn into useful and profitable diagnostic tests. But with an increasing range of new approaches come the first steps of progress. MPMx, in a $70 million alliance with Becton Dickinson & Co., is looking for differential expression in DNA, RNA, and proteins to identify relevant markers. In 2001 it received a patent on a gene related to metastatic melanoma, which it hopes will help identify patients with, or at risk of, the disease. Its series of markers for ovarian cancer (a far bigger market, particularly as ovarian cancer is 85 percent curable if detected early) are still two to three years away from being made into a research test, however, and at least another two from FDA approval.

Amplistar claims to have found a biomarker for ovarian cancer, which could be turned into an early-stage test by 2004. Their focus is not with genes but with the body's immunology, looking for cancer-specific antibodies produced as part of the body's natural immune response to cancer.

Other companies are focusing on very precise areas. Scientists at Minerva have found a specific part of the DNA-copying machinery they think is cancer specific. They will use this to develop both tissue-based and blood tests for early-stage cancers.

Cell Works Inc., as its name suggests, is working at the cellular, rather than molecular, level and has developed a way of finding and characterizing tumor cells—micrometastases—in blood. The company already has tests for prostate and breast cancer, and like most others, has plans to explore the link between diagnostics and therapeutics.

Ampersand Medical Corp. has developed a screening system for cervical cancer, which it hopes will improve on the traditional Pap smear. The company combines biomolecular markers with a novel sample-collection procedure in a system that could potentially enable point-of-care diagnosis of cervical cancer. The company is taking a similar approach to a test for ovarian cancer.

Commercializing their improved diagnostic tests is the next challenge for diagnostics companies. There can be long delays before a test is widely accepted and becomes valuable. PSA took several years, and HercepTest took off only after Herceptin was approved. Companies also have to figure out whether they want to go for a speedy market acceptance, in which case they must develop a relatively simple assay format and price the test in accordance with its initial reimbursement. Or they can start with a more complex test, convince the world of its value and justifiably high price, and then simplify it once it has become established. The strategy any company chooses will depend on how much financial elbow room it has.

New initiatives in the search for reliable diagnostic tests mean we are likely, over the next few years, to see a series of new and improved screening, diagnostic, and monitoring tests for cancer. The goal would be a panel of markers that are more accurate than those we have today.

MONITORING PROSTATE CANCER

Prostate-specific antigen (PSA) has emerged as the most important tumor marker to date for the diagnosis and clinical management of prostate cancer in men. But it's important to understand that PSA is organ specific, not cancer specific! This means that because the PSA protein is not specific to cancer (levels are high in other conditions such as prostatitis and benign prostatic hyperplasia, or BPH), it has a high false positive rate. Just because someone has a high PSA result, that doesn't mean that the person has cancer.

A digital rectal exam (DRE) and a serum prostate-specific antigen (PSA) test are both recommended for men who present to their physician with lower urinary tract symptoms, and all men over 50 years old.

"BPH and prostate cancer occur in men in about the same age groups, so when a man has a complaint about lower urinary tract symptoms, it is important for the physician to consider whether this man should be tested in some way for prostate cancer," said Michael Brawer, M.D., director of the Northwest Prostate Institute, Seattle, and chair of the Consultation's committee on "Detection of prostate cancer in a patient with BPH."

If either the PSA or the DRE produces results that suggest prostate cancer, a biopsy would be the next step. Indications for a biopsy would mean a PSA greater than 4.0 nanograms pre milliliter (ng/ml). A transurethral ultrasound-guided biopsy of the prostate's peripheral zone is the preferred method of biopsy, taking at least six systematic biopsy cores.

While screening seems to identify cancers confined to the prostate in the early stages, there is doubt whether screening can identify these tumors early enough to alter current mortality, because it is not possible to predict which microscopic tumors could be fatal. Screening aims to detect confined prostate tumors that can be removed. Screening can detect both untreatable and nonfatal tumors, as well as leaving an unknown number undetected.

There is some evidence that radical treatment of organ-confined cancer can lead to a small increase in long-term survival. Molecular markers of progression may lead to "watchful waiting" among men at low risk, but also may help men at higher risk who might benefit from major medical intervention.

In newly diagnosed patients the PSA level is proportional to the clinical stage of disease. Increasing PSA values correlate with an increasing Gleason score, a measure of the extent of the disease. An increase in the PSA value generally correlates with advancing tumor stage. Increasing PSA values after radiation therapy for localized prostate cancer or after radical prostatectomy often predict the development of metastases.

After the initiation of hormone therapy for metastatic disease, PSA can decline to normal values. The persistence of the decrease may predict a favorable response to therapy.

The decrease in serum PSA to undetectable levels following radical prostatectomy is an indicator of the success of surgery, just as a relapse is signaled by a subsequent increase in PSA levels.

MONITORING BREAST CANCER

Most cancer diagnostic tests are used, not for screening, but in order to monitor treatment. The benefits in linking diagnostic tests with particular therapies are exemplified in Dako AS's HercepTest. HER2/neu is the protein that is the target of Herceptin, a genetically engineered drug developed by Genentech. Most women who have breast cancer and are told they have high levels of HER2/neu, a protein receptor on the cell, would be unhappy to hear the news. Patients and doctors have come to understand that HER2/neu overexpression means they have a cancer that is likely to recur and spread. But Herceptin blocks the protein receptor and has been shown to increase survival among patients with advanced breast cancer. (See Chapter 6 for more about Herceptin.)

Routine follow-up care should include periodic blood testing for the CA125 marker. There is also a new tumor marker for breast cancer—CA27-29—to detect the progression of Stage II and III breast cancer.

After you are treated for breast cancer, your doctor should recommend follow-up mammographies every three months in the first year, every six months for the next two years, and annually after that. An annual mammogram is mandatory for all women by the age of 50, but women at higher risk should begin by the age of 40. Women with a family history of breast cancer should probably begin in their twenties.

There are new mammography techniques being developed, such as digital mammography, that will make the screening process less painful and more accurate.

A physical examination for lumps or other changes in the breast, along with a mammogram, ultrasound, and magnetic resonance imaging (MRI), can pinpoint the cancer. Fluid or cells from a lump can be withdrawn by needle aspiration for closer study. In a stereotactic breast biopsy, mammograms taken from various angles are used to determine the exact location of a suspicious area so a needle can be inserted to remove a small amount of tissue. Wire localization, the use of a wire in conjunction with a mammogram, is used to locate the abnormality for biopsy. A surgical biopsy is the removal of the lump to determine whether or not it is malignant.

Sometimes a sentinel lymph node biopsy may be used by the surgeon to determine the level of lymph node involvement. A radioactive substance or dye is injected into the region of the tumor and is carried to the first (sentinel) lymph node to receive lymph from the tumor. If the sentinel node contains cancer, more lymph nodes will be removed. If the sentinel node is cancer free, further lymph node surgery is not needed. There is no difference in diagnosis or treatment of male breast cancer. However, male breast cancers are usually diagnosed after metastasis has already occurred.

BSE, or breast self-exam, is also an important monitoring system to do yourself once a month. It's best to do it at the same time every month.

MONITORING OVARIAN CANCER

CA125, the tumor marker associated with ovarian cancer, is good at indicating the presence of tumor tissue and therefore is used by doctors for monitoring therapy. The test isn't recommended for screening, nor are the values directly proportional to the extent of disease.

As in breast carcinoma, ovarian cancer response to hormonal agents has been strongly associated with estrogen and progesterone receptor levels. Recent studies have found that estrogen receptor is expressed in 57 percent of primary ovarian epithelial carcinoma specimens.

Why does the FDA approve the use of the CA125 blood test only for following ovarian cancer, after a woman already has it? Why couldn't it be used as a screening test to find ovarian cancer early so that most women who are diagnosed would be in the very curable early states? PSA, the blood test for prostate cancer, is used in this way. Men are encouraged to have the test once a year to find early, and curable, prostate disease. Why not screen women for ovarian cancer?

Scientists will tell you that the CA125 test is not absolutely specific to ovarian cancer. Of course, no blood test is absolutely specific for anything. I was talking to the head of the tumor marker program at Memorial Sloan-Kettering Cancer Center in New York. He pointed out that his lab has seen high blood levels of CA125 in men with breast cancer. Also, patients with advanced breast, liver, and even colon cancer have high levels of this marker in their blood. But that's rare. And besides, any unexpected elevation of CA125 in a person's blood is cause for concern and should be thoroughly followed up.

Now, here's another objection to the use of CA125 as a screening tool. Because of the rarity of the disease, the cost to find those 0.1 percent of patients would be high. But maybe that's not true. Fifty million women, almost half of the female population, and a good percentage of women between 20 and 60 have an annual Pap smear examination. So they are already in the doctor's office.

Each of these Pap smear exams is accompanied by a physical exam, and usually a blood test. The blood test usually monitors their glucose and hemoglobin. Why not do a CA125 test on each of these blood samples? The extra cost would be about $5. That's an extra $250 million a year to measure CA125. It could save the lives of 17,000 women a year by catching ovarian cancer very early.

MONITORING COLORECTAL CANCER

Colon cancer can be detected early. When polyps and early-stage colon cancers are found and removed, the cure rate is nearly

100 percent, so early diagnosis is vital. Some of the diagnostic tools used for colorectal cancer include a digital rectal exam; a fecal occult-blood test; flexible sigmoidoscopy, the use of a lighted tube to find polyps and cancer in the rectum and first two feet of the colon; a colon X-ray (barium enema); and colonoscopy, the use of a lighted tube to examine the entire colon. Computed tomography (CT) scans of the colon, also called virtual colonoscopies, are still in the experimental phase as a screening tool.

The vast majority of colon cancers are treatable if detected at an early stage. Although colon cancer is the number-two cancer killer in the United States, less than 40 percent of the adults who are eligible for screening actually get it. The American Cancer Society recommends colon cancer screening for anyone age 50 or older, and for younger people who have a family history of the disease. Fecal occult-blood testing annually significantly reduces deaths from colorectal cancer.

Virtual Colonoscopy

Many people fear colon cancer screening because the most effective screening tool, colonoscopy, is uncomfortable and invasive. A new study from San Francisco Veterans Affairs Medical Center (SFVAMC) shows that a faster, safer, and potentially more pleasant technique works just as well. The so-called virtual colonoscopy uses a computed tomography (CT) scan to search for precancerous polyps.

The new study compared the virtual technique to standard colonoscopy, which involves snaking a long tube-shaped camera through the length of the colon. The study was published in the June 2001 issue of the journal *Radiology*.

"Since this technique requires no anesthesia, has no risk of complications from perforation or bleeding, and may be better tolerated by patients, we hope that it will increase the number of people willing to come in for screening," said lead author Judy Yee, M.D., University of California at San Francisco (UCSF) assistant professor of radiology and chief of CT and gastrointestinal radiology at SFVAMC.

In addition to its effectiveness at discovering colon cancer, virtual colonoscopy can also detect diseases and problems in other organs. The CT scan creates an image of the entire lower abdominal area, so radiologists can find problems such as kidney cancer, aneurysms in the aorta, and even lung cancers near the bottom of the lungs.

Virtual colonoscopy is also faster for the patient than traditional screening. Whereas standard colonoscopy can take from 30 minutes to one hour, not including time required to recover from sedatives, the CT scan takes only a few minutes to complete.

As many as 600,000 individuals in the United States are under care following surgery for colorectal cancer. About half are at some risk for its recurrence, due either to a new primary tumor or to metastatic disease undiscovered from a prior operation.

The death rate from colorectal cancer has begun to decline somewhat in recent years, and the five-year survival rate has improved, probably as a result of more aggressive diagnosis and therapeutics. However, the number of cases diagnosed annually has not seen a commensurate decline, nor has the incidence of metastatic disease in patients thought cured at time of primary surgery:

- Fifteen to 20 percent of patients with colorectal cancer present with distant metastases.
- Twenty-five percent of patients with diagnosis of colorectal carcinoma will have synchronous hepatic metastases. In another 25 percent, hepatic metastases will develop during the follow-up period. The natural history of untreated metastatic colorectal cancer to the liver is dismal, with virtually no five-year survivors.
- In spite of having localized disease at operation, 30 to 40 percent of patients initially classified as Dukes' B will develop metastases.
- Fifty percent of patients who undergo curative resection develop local, regional, or widespread recurrence. These statistics have remained relatively constant over several decades despite improved methods of early diagnosis and surgical treatment.

- Extrahepatic disease, lymph node involvement, and the inability to resect all gross metastases to the liver are generally considered absolute contraindications to resection for cure. No significant improvement in median survival has been demonstrated in this patient population.

CEA Markers

If you have undergone potentially curative surgery followed by adjuvant radiation and chemotherapy, you should have close surveillance to detect early recurrence. A persistent rise in serum carcinoembryonic antigen (CEA) may be the earliest indicator of recurrent colorectal cancer following curative resection of primary tumors. This rise may precede overt disease by several months.

An isolated elevation of CEA is not an uncommon event, and exhaustive, expensive investigation frequently fails to reveal an obvious site of recurrent disease. CEA elevations are falsely present in 10 to 40 percent of patients routinely monitored following resection.

The surveillance program consists of several patient evaluations. Patients are generally followed every three months for the first year. At each visit, patients undergo a complete history and physical examination, and serum CEA levels and liver function tests (alkaline phosphatase, lactate dehydrogenase, serum aspartate transaminase, and total bilirubin) are obtained. A chest X-ray and colonoscopy are obtained every six months during the first year.

During the second year of surveillance, all of the above evaluations are performed every six months. Beginning with the third year of follow-up, evaluations are performed on a yearly basis. A computerized axial tomography (CAT) scan of the abdomen and pelvis is generally recommended preoperatively or immediately postoperatively as a baseline. It is not necessary to order CAT scans routinely during the surveillance period unless liver function tests or CEA levels become elevated and/or the patient complains of pelvic/perineal pain and a local-regional recurrence is suspected.

If CEA levels become abnormal at any time during surveillance, they are repeated in four weeks; if there is a serial rise in CEA levels, the patient undergoes full evaluation consisting of colonoscopy, abdominal/pelvic CAT scan, chest X-ray, and liver function tests. If these tests are normal, the patient is scheduled for a "second-look" laparoscopy.

MONITORING LUNG CANCER

Detecting lung cancer lesions early may now be possible, and may have an impact on survival. Currently, most lung cancer is detected in a late stage, when the survival rate is quite low. Through early detection, perhaps 100,000 lives could be saved each year in the United States. Clearly, the greatest current need for a new diagnostic test for cancer is in lung cancer.

Smokers account for the large majority of lung cancer cases, but not all. Some people who have never smoked get lung cancer. Indeed, most smokers don't get lung cancer. This is probably more a tribute to the resilience of the body's repair mechanisms than to the benign effects of smoking.

Detecting smaller lung tumors with newer technologies such as computer tomography (CT) scans will certainly improve outcome. The problem is that the smallest size nodule detectable by CT scan is close to 5 mm—like the dot at the end of this sentence. By the time a lesion has grown to 5 mm, or close to the detectable range of CT scan, the cancer is late in the biology of the disease. Small primary lung cancers metastasize to regional lymph nodes or distant sites early in the disease process, making early detection even more important.

IMPROVEMENTS IN DIAGNOSTIC IMAGING

In the last two decades of the 20th century, several new diagnostic imaging techniques revolutionized the practice of medicine, making it possible to image the entire human body in exquisite anatomical detail. Today, computed tomography (CT), magnetic resonance imaging (MRI), and ultrasonography are commonly used to detect abnormalities well before they produce any clinical signs or symptoms of disease. These three-dimensional images can help doctors make precise diagnoses and design the best treatment. Now we are challenged to refine these technologies to detect molecular changes in the body. We need to use these techniques in such a way that no discomfort or side effects will occur in any patient.

Digital detectors will likely replace X-ray film, and invasive procedures will be replaced by "virtual examinations." With high-performance computers and sophisticated graphics hardware we could combine many of these imaging techniques into a single coherent three-dimensional picture that could rotate, magnify, and pan images in a few seconds. Computers can also add color to correspond with different kinds of body tissue. These evolving capabilities are allowing doctors to determine whether a tumor has invaded nearby organs or has grown around blood vessels.

The **conventional X-ray** is an old standby that is good for looking at bones. Contrast agents injected into your body enhance images and see tissue that would otherwise be invisible. Barium and iodine are two that are widely used.

A **computed tomography (CT)** scan moves around you to create several cross-sectional pictures, sort of like slices of a salami. The tissue resolution is much greater and more soft tissue differences can be distinguished, making it a better image for the chest than an X-ray.

Ultrasound is still a good way to tell the difference between a tumor and a cyst. High-frequency sound is directed into the body and reflected back from heat generated in the tissues. This test creates an image. This plays a key role in detection and characterization of tumors in soft tissues, including the ovary, testis, uterus, and prostate. It is also widely used to detect tumors in the abdomen, breast, and thyroid.

Images produced by MRI are the result of radio signals emitted by specific atoms in a patient who is lying in a strong magnetic field. MRI has been quite successful in scanning brains and spinal cords. It can also be used to image the heart and spine, the knee, bone marrow, cartilage, cerebrospinal and synovial fluid, and the abdomen. MRI may prove useful in imaging dense breast tissue, which is difficult to image with mammography, and is being used to guide needle biopsies.

SPECT (single photon emission computed tomography) images are created by detecting high-energy photons (gamma rays) that are produced by man-made radioactive atoms injected into the patient. The radioactive atoms can be used by themselves or by chemically tagging them to natural substances. They provide a means of investigating metabolic and physiologic processes. The most commonly used radioactive atom for SPECT is technetium-99. It has a half-life of six hours and can be linked to a variety of compounds for scanning various organs such as organic phosphate for bone scans; albumin for lung scans; and sulfur compound for liver, spleen, and bone marrow scans. SPECT can provide both anatomical information, such as the site of metastases of tumors, and functional information about blood flow and cell metabolism. Because of limited resolution, however, neither bones nor organs can be shown directly, or in the detail now available through CT or MRI.

One of the fastest-growing areas in clinical research is the use of PET (positron emission tomography) scan. Both PET and SPECT are unique in showing physiologic and biochemical processes whereas images from CT or MRI generally show morphology or structure. Like SPECT, PET images are created by detecting gamma rays produced by man-made radioactive atoms injected into the patient. These substances concentrate in different parts of the body. To generate PET images, short-lived (less than two hours) positron-emitting atoms are injected into the patient. When positrons travel short distances in tissues, they collide with nearby electrons and create two gamma rays that travel in opposite directions. The pair of rays can be picked up by gamma detectors surrounding the patient. This data are then processed by computer into a three-dimensional image.

The most common positron emitter is fluorine-18, which is used to label deoxyglucose, a form of glucose. Because most tumors metabolize glucose at a faster rate than does normal tissue, PET gamma detectors can pinpoint the site of tumor metastases. PET is frequently used in oncology today to characterize tumors, stage tumors, evaluate the extent of the disease, distinguish recurrent disease from treatment effects, and monitor therapy. With unlimited potential for the development of new tracers, PET has a promising future.

RISK FOR DEVELOPING CANCER

Everyone is at risk for developing cancer, so it is important to understand the kind of risk you may face. Fewer than 5 percent of cancer deaths are from heredity, but those inherited gene mutations are associated with a very high risk of cancer. Inherited *physiological* traits, however, do contribute to most cancers. For example, if you inherit fair skin, you are more prone to skin cancer. But if you protect your skin from extensive exposure to sunlight, an environmental carcinogen, you lower your risk considerably. In the same way, some people may inherit an inability to eliminate a certain carcinogen effectively. Only repeated exposure to that carcinogen will result in cancer.

Relative risk measures the number of risk factors you may face. It compares your risk with a certain exposure or trait to the risk for people who do not have that exposure or trait. If you smoke, for example, you are ten times more likely to develop lung cancer than a nonsmoker. Your relative risk is high.

Your lifetime risk is the probability that you will develop cancer or die from it over the course of your lifetime. If you are a man in the United States, you have a one in two lifetime risk of developing cancer, and if you are a woman, your risk is one in three. Eastern European men, including Russians, seem to have the highest risk of dying of cancer, with 205 deaths per 100,000 population. Women in Northern Europe are at highest risk, with 125 deaths per 100,000. For both men and women, the risk of being diagnosed with cancer is highest in North America.

Differences in cancer rates among races may also be traced to diet, lifestyle, and other factors in the environment. For example, Japanese women in Japan have one-fourth the risk of breast cancer that white women in the United States have. However, third-generation Japanese-American women have almost the same rate as other American women.

Cancer used to be a death sentence, but that's no longer true. In the beginning of the 20th century, few cancer patients could hope for survival. By the 1930s, about one in four survived for at least five years after treatment. By the end of the century, that survival rate was four out of ten.

The death rate has been declining since 1998, according to the Centers for Disease Control. Some types of cancer have very high survival rates. Localized breast cancer, for example, now has a survival rate of 97 percent compared to only 72 percent in the 1940s. Survival from acute lymphocytic leukemia went from 38 percent in the 1970s to 55 percent a decade later. The survival rate for prostate cancer increased from 67 to 93 percent in 20 years. Early detection is one of the reasons, as well as improved treatment that includes more effective prescription drugs.

And while the death rate is declining, the actual number of people dying is increasing because of the population growth and longer life expectancy. The cancer rate is growing faster than the population rate. The growth rate for cancer worldwide is 2.1 percent per year and the population growth is 1.7 percent a year. But, thank goodness, the death rates from some of these diseases stopped increasing in this country around 1992, and now they are beginning to decline slightly. Dr. Phillip Laszlo of the American Cancer Society tells us that death rates are already decreasing in prostate, breast, and lung cancers. It is expected that 60 percent of the people diagnosed with cancer every year will survive the disease.

Lung cancer is the leading cause of cancer death for both men and women in the United States, followed by prostate cancer for men and breast cancer for women. The third leading cause of death by cancer is cancer of the colon and rectum.

THE RISK OF AGE

The average life expectancy of both men and women in the United States is 74. This is the good news, since at the beginning of the 20th century it was only 47 years. The reverse of that is that the graying of America means that 115 million Americans are in the cancer-prone years of life. The longer you live, the more vulnerable you are to some cellular mishap. The incidence of cancer increases dramatically with age. Eighty-five percent of the 1.3 million diagnosed cancers each year occur in people over 50. Over the age of 65, you have a ten-times-greater risk of dying from cancer than those under 65, and rates of lung cancer, breast cancer, and prostate cancer are going up for older Americans.

RISK FACTORS YOU CAN CONTROL

In addition to genetic susceptibility and the natural aging process, we are all exposed to outside factors that contribute to our overall risk of getting cancer. Naturally, the more of these risk factors we have in our lives, the greater is our risk of getting cancer. Except for the environmental toxins and viruses, we can eliminate most of these risk factors from our lives.

Tobacco Smoking

Smoking tobacco accounts for 87 percent of lung cancers and is associated with cancers of the mouth, pharynx, larynx, esophagus, pancreas, uterus, cervix, kidney, and bladder. Secondhand smoke is also a carcinogen. Smoking is responsible for 30 percent of all cancer deaths in the United States yet is the most preventable cause of death. And living with a smoker is risky, too. Each year 3,000 nonsmoking adults die from lung cancer as a result of breathing secondhand smoke. Add drinking to the smoking picture and you create a volatile combination. Smoking and drinking creates a cancer risk that is greater than the sum of smoking or drinking taken separately. The combination also causes mouth, esophageal, and larynx cancers.

Diet and Nutrition

Improper diet and nutrition can be blamed for another third of all cancer deaths in the United States, according to the NCI. The risk is not only the types of foods you eat, but the way they are prepared, the size of the portions, the variety of foods in your diet, and the overall caloric balance. Animal (saturated) fats and red meat, in particular, are associated strongly with cancer of the colon and rectum. Saturated fats have also been implicated in prostate cancer. Salt seems to be a contributor to cancer of the stomach. Drinking very hot beverages increases the risk of esophageal cancer. You can lower your risk of cancer by eating more fruits, vegetables, and grains and less meat, dairy, and other high-fat foods. Balancing how much you eat with how much exercise you do will also lower your risk.

Ultraviolet B

Overexposure to the sun, most specifically to the higher-frequency ultraviolet B rays, is the cause of 90 percent of skin cancers, including melanomas. Some researchers now believe that childhood sunburns are more responsible for cancer than accumulated exposure to the sun. If you tan easily and don't burn, you are at much less risk.

Environmental and Chemical Toxins

Radon is a colorless, odorless, radioactive gas that seeps out of the earth. It has caused lung cancer in miners who work underground but is not considered a significant cause of cancer in the general population. Nevertheless, anyone building a house over a possible radon site is urged to get their home tested for the presence of this gas.

If you work around asbestos, benzene, diesel exhaust, formalde-hyde, or other **chemical toxins,** you are exposed to carcinogens that can cause cancer. These hazardous materials generally cause cancer of the lung, skin, bladder, and blood-forming systems. The good news is that finally, after many people have gotten cancer, there are strict controls on these hazardous materials in the United States. Occupational exposure to hazardous materials currently ac-counts for less than 5 percent of all cancer deaths.

Environmental pollutants—that is, pollutants in the air, water, and soil—may contribute to about 2 percent of fatal cancers, par-ticularly cancers of the lung and bladder. Diesel exhaust is a serious problem in large cities with bus and truck traffic. There is no con-clusive evidence that living near a toxic waste site or contaminated well causes cancer, yet this is under study; there is plenty of anec-dotal evidence to fuel the fire, as we have seen in recent books and movies like *A Civil Action* and *Erin Brockovich*.

Medications

About 1 percent of cancers can be blamed on medical products and procedures, but in general, the benefits outweigh the risks, as is the case with chemotherapy and radiation therapy. Some chemotherapy drugs can cause acute leukemia and even bladder cancer. Lymphomas can result from taking drugs that suppress the immune system. Estrogen replacement therapy, frequently used to treat symptoms of menopause, has been implicated in endometrial and breast cancer. Steroids have been linked to liver cancer. Other drugs currently under investigation as possible carcinogens in-clude tamoxifen, some fertility drugs, growth hormones, diuretics, and some cholesterol-lowering drugs. Oral contraceptives may in-crease the chance of liver tumors and premenopausal breast can-cer somewhat but may reduce the risk of ovarian, endometrial, and colorectal cancer.

Bacteria and DNA Viruses

The DNA viruses are the most common cancer-causing pathogens. They invade the host's cells and use the cells' DNA-synthesizing and protein-producing processes to clone themselves. The most important carcinogenic agents of this type are human papillomaviruses (types 16 and 18), which are transmitted sexually, and hepatitis B virus. The papillomaviruses can lead to cervical and other cancers. The hepatitis B virus can lead to liver cancer.

The Epstein-Barr virus is responsible for mononucleosis. Worldwide, it is a contributing factor to about half of the cancers of the pharynx, 30 percent of the cases of Hodgkin's disease, 10 percent of the cases of non-Hodgkin's lymphoma, and some gastric cancers.

The human immunodeficiency virus (HIV) can cause lymphoma and the soft-tissue cancer known as Kaposi's sarcoma.

The bacterium *Helicobacter pylori* causes stomach ulcers that can, in turn, lead to stomach cancer.

CONCLUSION

The new generation of drugs is a virtual medicine cabinet. We hope that there will be many uses of this new approach to treating cancer. These treatments target metabolic abnormalities that occur across a wide variety of cancers, and as you know, there are many cancers. It's not just one disease.

It is possible that these new drugs will stop many cancers from progressing. This kind of research will cross over into most forms of disease, like diabetes, Alzheimer's disease, and many forms of heart disease. The methodology of drug discovery tries to identify targets that are involved in disease. Anything that can be learned about those processes can be helpful in many types of disease.

The new cancer drugs can now treat cancer more like a chronic disease. The treatments will probably be taken for a long time, perhaps for life. This will add a whole new approach to those cancers that are now incurable.

Your options broaden enormously when you get into clinical trials, especially the well-designed trials that provide state-of-the-art care. First, go to an oncologist who is well trained and is expert in the field. This is the most important step. If an oncologist is part of a major designated investigator group of the National Institutes of Health, so much the better. A second opinion from a person in a designated cancer research investigation group would also be good as a referral.

With so much change occurring so quickly in medical science, it is important that you remain well informed about the latest ways to detect cancer—recurring cancer or a new cancer. Cancer, which is many diseases, is no longer an automatic death sentence. Today there are more than 10 million cancer survivors in America. More people survive cancer than die from it. This is due to early detection as well as improved treatment and better clinical management. But the management of your cancer is primarily up to you.

Speak up for your right to information about clinical trials and your right to the best possible treatment. As an informed patient and survivor, you can help others. The more you do for your own care, the more you do for all others. Here's one place to start fighting for more patient rights: Medicare does not cover the use of drugs taken orally, which is the way many of the new drugs are taken.

Remember what Dr. Vincent DiVita, director of the Yale Cancer Center, said on the *Charlie Rose Show:* "If your doctor tells you, 'There's nothing I can do for you,' don't believe it. There's almost always something we can do. You should take advantage of everything you can, because things are moving, and there's hope."

APPENDIX A

▼

NCI-DESIGNATED CANCER CENTERS

State	Name of Center
Alabama	UAB Comprehensive Cancer Center University of Alabama at Birmingham Birmingham
Arizona	Arizona Cancer Center University of Arizona Tucson
California	Cancer Research Center Beckman Research Institute, City of Hope Duarte Cancer Center Salk Institute La Jolla The Burnham Institute La Jolla

UCSD Cancer Center
University of California at San Diego
La Jolla

Jonsson Comprehensive Cancer Center
University of California at Los Angeles
Los Angeles

USC/Norris Comprehensive Cancer
Center
University of Southern California
Los Angeles

Chao Family Comprehensive Cancer
Center
University of Southern California at Irvine
Orange

UCSF Cancer Center and Cancer Re-
search Institute
University of California at San Francisco
San Francisco

Colorado   University of Colorado Cancer Center
                           University of Colorado Health Science
                           Center
                           Denver

Connecticut   Yale Cancer Center
                           Yale University School of Medicine
                           New Haven

District of   Lombardi Cancer Research Center
Columbia   Georgetown University Medical Center
                           Washington, DC

Florida	H. Lee Moffitt Cancer Center and Research Institute University of South Florida Tampa
Hawaii	Cancer Research Center of Hawaii University of Hawaii at Manoa Honolulu
Illinois	Cancer Research Center University of Chicago Cancer Research Center Chicago
	Robert H. Lurie Cancer Center Northwestern University Chicago
Indiana	Purdue University Cancer Center West Lafayette
	Indiana University Cancer Center Indianapolis
Iowa	University of Iowa Cancer Center Iowa City
Maine	The Jackson Laboratory Bar Harbor
Maryland	Johns Hopkins Oncology Center Baltimore
Massachusetts	Dana-Farber/Harvard Cancer Center Dana-Farber Cancer Institute Boston

Center for Cancer Research
Massachusetts Institute of Technology
Cambridge

Michigan   Comprehensive Cancer Center
University of Michigan
Ann Arbor

Barbara Ann Karmanos Cancer Institute
Wayne State University
    Operating the Meyer L. Prentis
    Comprehensive Cancer Center of Metro-
    politan Detroit
Detroit

Minnesota   University of Minnesota Cancer Center
Minneapolis

Mayo Clinic Cancer Center
Mayo Foundation
Rochester

Nebraska   University of Nebraska Medical Center/
Eppley Cancer Center
Omaha

New Hampshire   Norris Cotton Cancer Center
Dartmouth-Hitchcock Medical Center
Lebanon

New Jersey   The Cancer Institute of New Jersey
Robert Wood Johnson Medical School
New Brunswick

New York   Cancer Research Center
Albert Einstein College of Medicine
Bronx

Roswell Park Cancer Institute
Buffalo

Cold Spring Harbor Laboratory
Cold Spring Harbor

Kaplan Cancer Center
New York University Medical Center
New York

Memorial Sloan-Kettering Cancer Center
New York

American Health Foundation
New York

Herbert Irving Comprehensive Cancer
Center
College of Physicians and Surgeons
Columbia University
New York

North Carolina   UNC Lineberger Comprehensive Cancer
Center
University of North Carolina Chapel Hill
Chapel Hill

Duke Comprehensive Cancer Center
Duke University Medical Center
Durham

Comprehensive Cancer Center
Wake Forest University
Bowman Gray School of Medicine
Winston-Salem

Ohio	Case Western Reserve University and University Hospitals of Cleveland Cleveland
	Comprehensive Cancer Center Arthur G. James Cancer Hospital & Richard J. Solove Research Institute Ohio State University Columbus
Oregon	Oregon Cancer Center Oregon Health Sciences University Portland
Pennsylvania	University of Pennsylvania Cancer Center Philadelphia
	The Wistar Institute Philadelphia
	Fox Chase Cancer Center Philadelphia
	Kimmel Cancer Center Thomas Jefferson University Philadelphia
	University of Pittsburgh Cancer Institute Pittsburgh
Tennessee	St. Jude Children's Research Hospital Memphis
	Vanderbilt Cancer Center Vanderbilt University Nashville

Texas	University of Texas M. D. Anderson Cancer Center Houston
	San Antonio Cancer Institute San Antonio
Utah	Huntsman Cancer Institute University of Utah Salt Lake City
Vermont	Vermont Cancer Center University of Vermont Burlington
Virginia	Cancer Center University of Virginia, Health Sciences Center Charlottesville
	Massey Cancer Center Virginia Commonwealth University Richmond
Washington	Fred Hutchinson Cancer Research Center Seattle
	Wisconsin Comprehensive Cancer Center University of Wisconsin Madison
	McArdle Laboratory for Cancer Research University of Wisconsin Madison

Source: National Cancer Institute

APPENDIX B

▼

CANCER INFORMATION RESOURCES

GENERAL CANCER INFORMATION

American Cancer Society
http://www.cancer.org
    Web site of the nationwide, community-based, voluntary health organization dedicated to eliminating cancer as a major health problem by preventing cancer, saving lives, and diminishing suffering from cancer through research, education, advocacy, and service.

Cancer Care
http://www.cancercareinc.org
    Web site of the oldest (1944) and largest national nonprofit agency providing emotional support, information, and practical help to people with cancer and their loved ones.

Cancer Information Network
http://www.cancernetwork.com
    Professional information service for medical people involved in the care and treatment of patients with cancer.

Cancer Survivors' Network
http://cancersurvivorsnetwork.org
Source of information and support for cancer patients and their loved ones provided by the American Cancer Society.

Cancer Trials
http://www.cancernet.nci.nih.gov
Comprehensive clinical trial information for patients, healthcare professionals, and the public.

CancerLinks
http://www.cancerlinks.org
Site designed to make searching the World Wide Web for information about cancer faster and easier.

CancerLinksUSA
http://www.cancerlinksusa.com
Noncommercial site founded to provide support and information to cancer patients and their caregivers.

CancerNet
http://www.cancernet.nci.nih.gov
Recent and accurate cancer information from the National Cancer Institute and access to CancerLit, a bibliographic database.

Corporate Angel Network (CAN)
http://www.corpangelnetwork.org
This organization provides cancer patients with free air transportation to and from medical facilities using empty seats on corporate aircraft. Patients must meet CAN's qualifications but do not need to meet any financial need criteria.

InteliHealth
http://www.intelihealth.com
A health information company founded in 1996 that is a joint venture of Aetna U.S. Healthcare and Johns Hopkins University and Health System.

M. D. Anderson Cancer Center, University of Texas
http://www.mdanderson.org
Web site of one of the National Cancer Institute's designated Comprehensive Cancer Centers focused exclusively on cancer patient care, research, education, and prevention

Mayo Clinic Health Oasis
http://www.mayohealth.org
A source of health information from the Mayo Clinic that includes a Cancer Center.

Memorial Sloan-Kettering Cancer Center
http://www.mskcc.org
Web site of the world's oldest and largest private institution (established in 1884) devoted to prevention, patient care, research, and education in cancer.

National Cancer Institute
http://www.nci.nih.gov
Information about the institute and its programs.

OncoLink of the University of Pennsylvania
http://cancer.med.upenn.edu
Founded in 1994 by Penn cancer specialists with a mission to help cancer patients, families, health-care professionals, and the general public get accurate cancer-related information at no charge.

Pharmaceutical Research and Manufacturers of America (PhRMA)
http://www.phrma.org
PhRMA represents about 100 U.S. companies that have a primary commitment to pharmaceutical research.

Women's Cancer Network
http://www.wcn.org
Site developed by the Gynecologic Cancer Foundation and dedicated to informing women around the world about gynecologic cancer.

PEDIATRIC CANCER INFORMATION

The Pediatric Cancer Care Network is a collaboration between two NCI-sponsored cooperative groups that study children's cancers and the Blue Cross and Blue Shield Association. The network's purpose is to ensure that children of Blue Cross and Blue Shield subscribers receive care at designated centers of cancer excellence. The web sites of Blue Cross and Blue Shield, Candlelighters, and National Childhood Cancer Foundation, listed here, compose this network.

Blue Cross and Blue Shield Caring Program for Children
www.bluecares.com/blue/kids
This web site has information on the program and contains links to participating plans, as well as news about diseases affecting children.

Candlelighters Childhood Cancer Foundation (CCCF)
www.candlelighters.org
This site is an introduction to the programs and services of CCCF including publications and local chapters. CCCF is an international nonprofit organization dedicated to educating, supporting, serving, and advocating for families of children with cancer, survivors of childhood cancer, and the professionals who care for them.

Children's Cancer Research Fund
www.ccrf.org
Its goal is to establish and foster research in childhood cancer, as well as enrich the quality of life for children with cancer by improving clinical and support services.

National Childhood Cancer Foundation/Children's Cancer Group (NCCF/CCG)
www.nccf.org
Information about the facts of childhood cancer, stories of cancer survivors, clinical trial information on Children's Cancer

Group, and locations of CCG institutions. A separate password-protected area is maintained for CCG membership. This area contains detailed CCG protocols, group operational information, and group collaboration services such as group-specific mailing lists and a web-based conference board.

Widen the Web
www.sunsite.unc.edu/hcrl/
This site provides a forum for children who have survived cancer to share ideas and insight about surviving cancer with peers.

CANCER-RELATED JOURNALS ON-LINE

There are over 150 cancer-related journals currently on-line, including:

Acta Haematologica
Acta Oncologica
American Journal of Clinical Oncology
American Journal of Hematology
American Journal of Pathology: Journal of the American Society of Investigative Pathology
Angiogenesis
Angiogenesis Research
Annals of Oncology
Annals of Surgical Oncology
Anti-Cancer Drug Design
Anti-Cancer Drugs
Antimicrobial Agents and Chemotherapy
Apoptosis
BBA: Biochimica et Biophysica Acta
Biotherapy
Blood: Journal of the American Society of Hematology
Blood Cells, Molecules, and Diseases (e-mail journal)
Blood Weekly
BMJ: British Medical Journal

Bone Marrow Transplantation
Brain Tumor Pathology
Breast Cancer Research
Breast Cancer Research and Treatment
British Journal of Cancer
British Journal of Haematology
CA: A Cancer Journal for Clinicians
Cancer: Journal of the American Cancer Society
Cancer and Metastasis Reviews
Cancer Biochemistry Biophysics
Cancer Biotechnology Weekly
Cancer Biotherapy and Radio-pharmaceuticals
Cancer Case Presentations: The Tumor Board
Cancer Causes and Control
Cancer Chemotherapy and Pharmacology
Cancer Control: Journal of the Moffitt Cancer Center
Cancer Cytopathology
Cancer Detection and Prevention
Cancer Epidemiology Biomarkers & Prevention
Cancer Gene Therapy
Cancer Genetics and Cytogenetics
Cancer Immunology, Immunotherapy
Cancer Journal, The
Cancer Letters
Cancer Pain Reviews
Cancer Practice
Cancer Prevention and Control
Cancer Research
Cancer Research, Therapy and Control
Cancer Strategy
Cancer Treatment Reviews
Cancer Weekly Plus
Cancer/Radiothérapie
Carcinogenesis
Cell Online
Chemotherapie Journal
Chemotherapy

Clinical and Experimental Metastasis
Clinical Cancer Research
Clinical Oncology
Critical Reviews in Oncogenesis
Current Advances in Cancer Research
Current Opinion in Hematology
Current Opinion in Oncology
Current Problems in Cancer
Curriculum Oncologicum
Electronic Journal of Oncology
European Cancer News
European Journal of Cancer
European Journal of Cancer Care
European Journal of Cancer Prevention
European Journal of Surgical Oncology
Experimental Hematology
Frontiers in Bioscience
Genes, Chromosomes, and Cancer
GI Cancer
Gynecologic Oncology
Haemotologica, Journal of Hematology On-Line
Hematological Oncology
Hematology
Hematology/Oncology Clinics of North America
IDEAL (On-line scientific journal library; over 170 journals)
International Journal of Cancer
International Journal of Gynecological Cancer
International Journal of Pediatric Hematology and Oncology
International Journal of Radiation Biology
International Journal of Radiation Oncology Biology Physics
Internet Oncology Discussion Groups (compiled by the University
   of Pennsylvania OncoLink service)
Invasion and Metastasis
Investigational New Drugs: The Journal of New Anticancer Agents
Japanese Journal of Cancer Research
Japanese Journal of Clinical Oncology Online
JAMA: Journal of the American Medical Association

JAMA's Cancer-Related Abstracts
JNCI: Journal of the National Cancer Institute
Journal of Cancer Research and Clinical Oncology
Journal of Clinical Investigation
Journal of Clinical Oncology: Journal of the American Society of Clinical Oncology
Journal of Environmental Pathology, Toxicology and Oncology
Journal of Experimental Therapeutics and Oncology
Journal of Image Guided Surgery
Journal of Immunotherapy
Journal of Neuro-Oncology
Journal of Oncology Pharmacy Practice
Journal of Pediatric Hematology/Oncology
Journal of Pediatric Oncology Nursing
Journal of Surgical Oncology
Lancet, The
Leukemia and Lymphoma
Leukemia Research
Lung Cancer
Medical and Pediatric Oncology
Medical Oncology
Medscape Oncology
Melanoma Research
Molecular and Cellular Biochemistry
Molecular Carcinogenesis
Mutagenesis
Nature
Nature Medicine
Neoplasia
Neoplasma
New England Journal of Medicine
Nutrition and Cancer
Oncogene
Oncology: International Journal of Cancer Research and Treatment
Oncology: Review
Oncology Issues
Oncology Times

Onkologe, Der
Onkologie
Oral Oncology
Pain Research and Management
Pathology and Oncology Research
Pediatric Hematology and Oncology
Pediatric Hematology/Oncology
Pharmacy World & Science
PNAS: Proceedings of the National Academy of Sciences
Proceedings of the American Association for Cancer Research
Proceedings of the American Society for Clinical Oncology
Prostate Cancer
Psycho-Oncology
Quality of Life Research
Radiation Oncology Investigations
Radiation Research
Radiotherapy and Oncology
Reviews on Cancer Online
Science: Journal of the American Association for the Advancement of Science
Sein, La
Seminars in Cancer Biology
Seminars in Oncology
Seminars in Radiation Oncology
Seminars in Surgical Oncology
Seminars in Urologic Oncology
Supportive Care in Cancer
Surgical Oncology
Surgical Oncology Clinics of North America
Teratogenesis, Carcinogenesis, and Mutagenesis
Tumor Biology
Tumor Targeting
Tumori
Urologic Oncology

APPENDIX C

▼

BIOTECH RESEARCH CENTERS

Aeterna Labs
1405 Parc-Technologique
Boulevard
Quebec G1P 4P5
Quebec, Canada
Telephone: 418-652-8525
Fax: 418-652-0881
Web site: www.aeterna.com

Aphton Corporation
444 Brickell Avenue
Suite 51-507
Miami, FL 33131
Telephone: 305-374-7338
Fax: 305-374-7615
Web site: www.aphton.com

AstraZeneca
15 Stanhope Gate
London W1K 1LN
United Kingdom

Telephone: 302-886-4065
Web site: www.astrazeneca.com

Biomira
2011 94th Street
Alberta T6N 1H1
Edmonton, Canada
Telephone: 780-450-3761
Fax: 780-463-0871
Web site: www.biomira.com

Bristol-Myers Squibb
345 Park Avenue
New York, NY 10154
Telephone: 212-546-4000
Fax: 212-546-4020
Web site: www.bristolmyers.com

Celgene Corporation
7 Powder Horn Drive
Warren, NJ 07059

Telephone: 732-271-1001
Fax: 732-271-4184
Web site: www.celgene.com

Cell Genesys
342 Lakeside Drive
Foster City, CA 94404
Telephone: 650-425-4400
Fax: 650-358-0803
Web site: www.cellgenesys.com

Cell Pathways
702 Electronic Drive
Horsham, PA 19044
Telephone: 215-706-3800
Fax: 215-706-3801
Web site: www.cellpathways.com

Chiron
4560 Horton Street
Emeryville, CA 94608
Telephone: 510-655-8730
Fax: 510-655-9910
Web site: www.chiron.com

Corixa
1124 Columbia Street
Suite 200
Seattle, WA 98104
Telephone: 206-754-5711
Fax: 206-754-5715
Web site: www.corixa.com

Dendreon
3005 First Avenue
Seattle, WA 98121
Telephone: 206-256-4545

Fax: 206-256-0571
Web site: www.dendreon.com

EntreMed
9640 Medical Center Drive
Suite 200
Rockville, MD 20850
Telephone: 301-217-9858
Fax: 301-217-9594
Web site: www.entremed.com

Geneara
5110 Campus Drive
Plymouth Meeting, PA 19462
Telephone: 610-941-4020
Fax: 610-941-5399

Genentech
One DNA Way
South San Francisco, CA 94080
Telephone: 650-225-1000
Fax: 650-225-6000
Web site: www.genentech.com

Genta Incorporated
2 Oak Way
Berkeley Heights, NJ 07922
Telephone: 908-286-3980
Fax: 908-464-1701
Web site: www.genta.com

Genzyme Corporation
One Kendall Square
Cambridge, MA 02139
Telephone: 617-252-7500
Fax: 617-494-6561

GlaxoSmithKline Beecham
Glaxo Wellcome House
Berkeley Avenue
Greenford, Middlesex UB6 ONN
United Kingdom
Telephone: 171-493-4060
Fax: 181-966-8330

ImClone Systems
180 Varick Street
New York, NY 10014
Telephone: 212-645-1405
Fax: 212-645-2054
Web site: www.imclone.com

Immunex
51 University Street
Seattle, WA 98101
Telephone: 206-587-0430
Fax: 206-587-0606
Web site: www.immunex.com

Immunomedics
300 American Road
Morris Plains, NJ 07950
Telephone: 973-605-8200
Fax: 973-605-8282
Web site:
www.immunomedics.com

Introgen Therapeutics, Inc.
301 Congress Avenue
Suite 1850
Austin, TX 78701
Telephone: 512-708-9310
Fax: 512-708-9311
Web site: www.introgen.com

Medarex
707 State Road #206
Princeton, NJ 08854
Telephone: 609-430-2880
Fax: 908-713-6002
E-mail: medarex@aol.com

NeoRx
410 West Harrison Street
Seattle, WA 98119
Telephone: 206-281-7001
Fax: 206-298-9442
Web site: www.neorx.com

Novartis
Lichtstrasse 35
CH-4002 Basel
Switzerland
Telephone: 908-522-6899
Fax: 908-522-6897
Web site:
www.group.novartis.com

Progenics Pharmaceuticals
777 Old Saw Mill River Road
Tarrytown, NY 10591
Telephone: 914-789-2800
Fax: 914-789-2817
Web site: www.progenics.com

Schering-Plough
Muellerstrasse 178
13353 Berlin
Germany
Telephone: 973-276-2164
Fax: 973-276-2005
Web site: www.schering.com

SciClone Pharmaceuticals
901 Mariner's Island Boulevard
Suite 205
San Mateo, CA 94404
Telephone: 650-358-3456
Fax: 650-358-3469
Web site: www.sciclone.com

Titan Pharmaceuticals
400 Oyster Point Boulevard
Suite 505
South San Francisco, CA 94080
Telephone: 650-244-4990
Fax: 650-244-4956
Web site: www.titanpharm.com

SuperGen
4140 Dublin Boulevard
Suite 200
Dublin, CA 94568
Telephone: 925-560-0100
Fax: 925-327-7347
Web site: www.supergen.com

INDEX

239

Hartmann, Lynn, 80–81
HDR (high dose rate) brachytherapy, for
    breast cancer, 75–76
Health-care team, 47–56
    cancer care centers, 50, 217–23
    doctors, hiring, 48–50
    information about treatments, 55–56
    putting together, 55
    type of help available for, 50–55
    your role on, 48
Health insurance
    clinical trials and, 42
    home health aides and, 53
    nurses and, 51
Heart failure, Myocet and, 66
Hellmann, Susan D., 62–63
Hematopoietic growth factors. *See*
    Colony-stimulating factors
Henney, Christopher S., 118
Hepatitis B virus, 213
HercepTest, 197, 199
Herceptin (trastuzumab), 23, 25, 142,
    197
    breast cancer and, 23, 58, 59–63, 199
    clinical trials, 86–87
    side effects, 61, 63
    Taxotere and, 68–69
    pancreatic cancer and, 156
Hereditary ovarian cancer, 95–96
Heredity, 208. *See also* Genes
    breast cancer and, 58, 76
    colon cancer and, 139
    pancreatic cancer and, 151
    skin cancer and, 208
HER2/neu gene, 15, 142, 150, 156
    breast cancer and, 58, 59–63, 195, 199
    clinical trials, 62, 87
    overexpression, 61–62, 199
Hexalen, ovarian cancer and, 92
HIV (human immunodeficiency virus),
    166, 213
HLA-B7 protein, melanoma and, 188
Hodgkin's disease, 165–66, 213
Holladay, Clinton T., 105
Holladay, David A., 105
Holmium-166 DOTMP, multiple
    myeloma and, 171–72
Home health aides, 53
Home hospice care, 54–55
Hormone therapy
    for breast cancer, 69–75, 83
        Arimidex, 72–73
        Aromasin, 73–74

        letrozole, 73
        tamoxifen, 69–72, 73, 74
        Zoladex, 74–75
    for prostate cancer, 108–11, 199
Hospice care, 54–55
Hospital social workers, 51–52
Howard Hughes Medical Institute,
    140–41
HPV16E6, ovarian cancer and, 98
HSP65, ovarian cancer and, 98
HSV-tk gene, prostate cancer and, 120
Human genome, xiv, 3–4, 10, 13. *See also*
    DNA
HuM291, lymphoma and, 175
Hu1D10, leukemia and, 175
Hybridomas, monoclonal antibodies
    and, 23–24

Ibandronate, multiple myeloma and, 172
IDEC Pharmaceuticals, 24, 25, 164–65,
    167
ILEX Oncology, 31–32
IMC-C225
    colon cancer and, 141–42
    lung cancer and, 136
ImClone Systems, 25, 136, 141–43, 237
IMC-1C11, colon cancer and, 142–43
Immune system, 10, 25–26
    breast cancer vaccine and, 63–64
    cancer cells and, 19–22
Immunomedics, 168, 237
Immunotherapy, 16, 22–30. *See also*
    Cytokines; Monoclonal antibodies
    therapy; Vaccines
    for esophageal cancer, 150
    for melanoma, 181–86
Indomethacin, colon cancer and, 147
Information sources, 55–56, 225–33
    breast cancer, 84–85
    for clinical trials, 42–44
    digestive system cancers, 151–52
    leukemia, 173–74
    lung cancer, 135–36
    lymphoma, 173–74
    melanoma, 189
    multiple myeloma, 173–74
    ovarian cancer, 96–97
    pediatric cancer, 228–29
    prostate cancer, 119–20
INGN201, lung cancer and, 131–32
Insurance companies. *See* Health insur-
    ance
InteliHealth, 226